SPECIAL HEART

A Journey of Faith, Hope, Courage and Love

BRET BAIER

WITH JIM MILLS

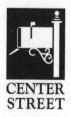

CENTER
STREET

New York Nashville Boston

Center Street
Hachette Book Group
237 Park Avenue
New York, NY 10017

www.CenterStreet.com

Printed in the United States of America

RRD-C

First Edition: June 2014
10 9 8 7 6 5 4 3 2 1

Center Street is a division of Hachette Book Group, Inc.
The Center Street name and logo are trademarks of Hachette Book Group, Inc.

The Hachette Speakers Bureau provides a wide range of authors for speaking events. To find out more, go to www.HachetteSpeakersBureau.com or call (866) 376-6591.

The publisher is not responsible for websites (or their content) that are not owned by the publisher.

Library of Congress Cataloging-in-Publication Data
Baier, Bret.
  Special heart : a journey of faith, hope, courage and love / Bret Baier with Jim Mills. -- First edition.
      pages cm
  ISBN 978-1-4555-8363-8 (hardback) -- ISBN 978-1-4555-8364-5 (ebook) -- ISBN 978-1-4789-0084-9 (audio download) 1. Baier, Bret. 2. Television journalists--United States--Biography. I. Title.
  PN4874.B235A3 2014
  070.4092--dc23
  [B]
                          2013048151

*For Amy—the most amazing wife and mother to
our children and my co-anchor in life.*

CONTENTS

PROLOGUE

Washington, D.C.—January 6, 2014—7:02 a.m.

It's Monday morning—the first full week of the New Year. After its traditional—and long—Christmas break, Capitol Hill is slowly coming back to life. As I approach the Fox News bureau two blocks from the U.S. Capitol, I look down at my watch and see I am running a few minutes late.

I am here early this morning so I can appear on several local Fox stations across the country—part of an affiliate outreach project I began about eight months ago. I really enjoy doing these affiliate interviews. Even though *Special Report* doesn't air for another eleven hours, mixing it up with anchors from coast to coast this early in the morning helps me get my head in the game for the rest of the day. It also gives me a golden opportunity to hear what stories might be resonating nationwide and worth paying attention to on tonight's show.

Under the banner "all politics is local," D.C., like much of the rest of the country, is being affected by what meteorologists are calling a *polar vortex*. It's a new phrase for me, but frankly, it seems like just a high-tech way of saying it's very cold outside. Fancy terminology or not, weather conditions across the country are get-

ting a lot of attention on all the networks as I enter the bureau and scan the bank of television monitors in the newsroom.

Despite the extreme temperatures, much about Washington seems quite normal this morning. Just six days into the New Year, the 2014 political cauldron is already starting to boil up as both parties jockey for tactical advantage in the November midterm elections—still a full ten months away. First out of the blocks on Capitol Hill is a measure to extend unemployment benefits; right behind that—an expected fight over raising the minimum wage. Based on political talking points unfurled on the Sunday talk shows, both sides seem quite comfortable hunkering down in their well-worn trenches for some traditional class warfare over income inequality—a topic President Obama has been talking a lot about lately.

New Jersey Republican Governor Chris Christie, frequently mentioned as a possible 2016 presidential contender, is facing questions this week over whether he intentionally created a traffic jam on the George Washington Bridge in order to punish a mayor who didn't support his re-election bid.

So-called *Bridgegate* has also become quite fertile ground for the late-night comics. Combined with the less-than-stellar rollout of President Obama's signature health care plan, it is safe to say stand-up comedians everywhere will have plenty of material to see them through the vortex and well into the spring.

With the Senate confirmation of a new Federal Reserve Chair, a Supreme Court hold on same-sex marriage in Utah, an emerging $1.1 trillion budget bill, an upcoming vote on raising the debt limit and the rise of al Qaeda in Iraq and this promises to be a very busy week.

As I sit at my computer checking the newswires, my assistant Katy Ricalde hands me the list of the affiliates I'll be talking with and the precise times they will come to me in the studio—the same studio we use for *Special Report* every night at 6:00 p.m. ET.

WTXF Philadelphia with Mike Jerrick and Sheinelle Jones at 7:30 a.m. WTVT Tampa with Russell Rhodes at 7:35 a.m. WAGA Atlanta with Gurvir Dhindsa at 7:40 a.m., followed by live hits spaced out every five minutes with Dave Froehlich at KTBC in Austin, John Brown at WOFL in Orlando, Greg Kelly and Rosanna Scotto at WNYW in New York City, Tom Butler at KMSP in Minneapolis, Tony McEwing at KTTV in Los Angeles, Allison Seymour at WTTG in Washington, D.C., Anqunette "Q" Jamison at WJBK in Detroit, Ernie Freeman at WHBQ in Memphis, Shannon Mulaire at WFXT in Boston, Tim Ryan and Lauren Przybyl at KDFW in Dallas, Natalie Bomke at WFLD in Chicago, and wrapping up with Jose Grinan at KRIV in Houston at 9:20 a.m.

Drop in a few live segments with *Fox & Friends* and *Happening Now* on Fox News Channel and a couple of radio hits with WLS in Chicago and *Kilmeade & Friends*, and my first day back following the break is proving to be extremely hectic—just the way I like it.

After I finish up the studio interviews, I walk through the newsroom and morning assignment desk coordinator, Pat Summers, greets me with a robust "Happy Anniversary!" It's hard for me to believe, but today is the fifth year anniversary of the day I started anchoring *Special Report*. Given the job when my friend and mentor Brit Hume stepped down from the anchor chair in January 2009, I am sure some critics were standing by

with egg timers to see how long I would last—especially filling the shoes of a broadcast legend like Brit. But 1,305 shows later, and I'm still here. Needless to say, anchoring *Special Report* the past five years has been the high point of my professional life. By all measurements the program is doing great—consistently one of the top four most-watched news shows in all of cable, number one in its time slot and picking up new viewers all the time.

As exciting and interesting as anchoring *Special Report* is, the daily challenge for me is that my world is dictated by the clock and that unforgiving second hand as it marches toward the moment right before show time when my stage manager, Mary Pat Dennert, holds up her hand and counts out *"Ten—Nine—Eight—Seven—Six..."* When Mary Pat gets to *"Five"*—everything in the studio—including Mary Pat—goes silent as she performs the rest of the count using only her fingers.

A few minutes before we go on the air each night I often catch myself glancing up at the clock I have been battling with all day as I try to regain a little non-TV-world perspective. I count the many blessings in my life—my beautiful and loving wife, Amy, and two wonderful sons, Paul and Daniel, who fill our lives with so much joy. Whether it's a father-son golf lesson that morphs into a sandcastle-making class in the practice bunker, or all three fully-costumed Baier boys—*me and the other two*—spending a Saturday bouncing around the house playing Batman and Robin; network news anchor or not—it doesn't get any better than that!

As the final seconds tick down tonight I am reminded that it wasn't too long ago when the clock on the wall had an entirely different meaning for me. Instead of

counting me down to host a television show or signaling me that it was time to race to the White House lawn to do a live shot, one day that second hand came to a screeching halt. It was June 30, 2007—the day I was confronted with the sobering reality that I was not in control of anything.

Throughout my career in journalism I always felt as if I could out-hustle the next guy and get to the bottom of whatever story I was assigned. I could always dig down, work hard and tackle the challenge before me. I always prided myself on being able to put my nose to the grindstone, work the problem, achieve the goal, make it happen—*all on deadline*. But not this time. I quickly learned that if I was going to be of any help to my family in its greatest moment of need I was going to have to reset my priorities, take a leap of faith and rely on a completely different set of resources than I was used to.

Mary Pat's silent countdown now at "*3...2...1*," the red light on top of the studio camera pops on and she signals me to start tonight's anniversary edition of *Special Report*.

"*Welcome to Washington. I'm Bret Baier...*"

It might be the standard, familiar introduction I use at the beginning of every show, but with tonight's fifth anniversary I have an extra measure of joy and thankfulness in my heart. I am also overflowing with gratefulness that the Baier family made it through the roughest part of the storm. But I think I might be getting a little ahead of myself...

SPECIAL HEART

CHAPTER ONE

Young Man on the Move

It was a beautiful, crystal clear day in Atlanta. The sticky heat of the summer was behind us, but we still had a few weeks to go before the full autumn chill would set in. The minute I woke up I remember thinking, "Man, if I didn't have to go into work today, this would be a perfect day to play some golf."

"Maybe I could finish up my story assignments early and still be able to hit a bucket of balls after work," I thought as I drove to the Fox News bureau near Georgia Tech. Anyone who knows me is well aware of my passion—some might say my obsession—with hitting that little white ball all over God's creation. And this glorious September morning was no exception.

Growing up nearby in the Atlanta suburbs, I played golf every chance I got at Dunwoody Country Club, conveniently located about a mile from my house. To be journalistically precise, that stretch of road from my house to Dunwoody was exactly 1.2 miles. It's a number I will never forget, because during the long summer days of my youth, I would walk it, run it, moped it,

and sometimes hitch rides on it to get back and forth to the golf course. Later, when I had my own car but little money for gas, I often begged the Saint of the Empty Gas Tank for precisely 1.2 miles' worth of heavenly fumes so I could make it home from Dunwoody late at night.

My first car, a 1982 green Ford Grenada, was affectionately nicknamed Kermit the Frog by my friends. With his forest-green exterior and emerald-green cloth interior, what Kermit lacked in style and class he made up for in character and originality. Multitalented, Kermit actually inspired a few original phrases around my neighborhood in those days. One was the "car blister" because of the way Kermit's interior roof cloth constantly drooped down and slapped passengers and driver upside the head as though they were in a 1970s' sparring match with Muhammad Ali. During typically muggy Atlanta summer days, anyone who drove with Kermit's windows wide open had better be prepared to go several rounds with no corner man to close the cuts.

Kermit was not exactly the textbook Casanova chariot a young man dreams about to impress potential high school sweethearts, so I was always thankful when autumn came and I could roll up the windows and keep all that head slapping to a minimum. I often drove Kermit, with no sweethearts anywhere to be found, to the Dunwoody chipping green late at night where I would park and strategically aim my high-beam lights just right so I could practice my short game well into the evening after everyone else had left for the day. Golf went way beyond a transitory childhood preoccupation for me. I played so much golf I eventually became one of the top

players on my high school team, which went on to win state finals my senior year.

Although I was totally dedicated to golf during high school, I did fit in a few other activities from time to time, such as being sports editor of the Marist School newspaper *The Blue & Gold*, interning for sportscaster Ernie Johnson Jr. at Atlanta's WSB television station, serving as president of the Marist student council, and something that never, ever seemed to make it onto my résumé reel over the years: playing the Cowardly Lion and Tevye in school productions of *The Wiz* and *Fiddler on the Roof*. The VHS tapes of those performances are hermetically sealed and under lock and key in an underground bunker somewhere in the mountains of West Virginia.

After high school I went on to DePauw University in Greencastle, Indiana, where I continued playing competitive golf at the NCAA level and double majored in Political Science and English. DePauw offered me a wonderful opportunity to combine the two great passions in my seventeen-year-old life—golf and journalism.

Sometimes I don't know how I fit it all in, but along with my class work, fraternity responsibilities, and active social life, I was playing some serious golf under the tutelage of Coach Ted Katula, who became a great influence on me during my college years. Coach Katula, or Katman as he was affectionately called, was a great athlete in his younger years, having played on both the Ohio State football team under Woody Hayes and the Ohio State golf team that included the great Jack Nicklaus.

A fantastic golfer, Katman was also a brilliant teacher

of golf—and life. He had a huge influence on everyone who had the good fortune to be coached by him. And that was a very long list. In fact, just a few months after I landed on campus, a former member of one of Katman's golf teams by the name of Quayle made some nationwide, nongolf news by getting himself elected vice president of the United States.

Often when we traveled to golf tournaments throughout the Midwest, Coach Katula, a wonderful storyteller, would regale us with unbelievable tales collected over decades of playing and coaching. But some of Katman's best stories came courtesy of his days in the 1960s when he served as DePauw's student activities director and was responsible for entertainment on campus.

With his winsome personality, sense of humor, and down-to-earth midwestern take on life, Katman was successful in cajoling some very big names to come to the relatively small DePauw campus to perform. Smokey Robinson, Billy Joel, the Byrds, and the Temptations were just a few of the acts he recruited. Once, in the mid 1960s, Katman booked the Isley Brothers for a concert, and they apparently blew the doors off the place—perhaps with a bit of an assist from the group's young, unknown guitar player, Jimi Hendrix.

For golf team road trips, Katman would typically start out very early in the morning in a large team van and pick up several of us in front of our fraternity house so we could get to tournament sites in plenty of time to play practice rounds before the actual match.

One early Saturday morning, making his stop at Sigma Chi, Katman arrived before a road trip that had been unmercifully scheduled right after a formal dance at the house the previous evening. Staying up all night

dancing and partying with my date, I completely lost track of time and Coach Katula's schedule to get the team on the road. The only way I could make it to the van and not miss the trip was to show up wearing my tuxedo. Doubled over in laughter, Katman said, "Baiersy, all my years being a coach here, this is a first! Even Dan Quayle never showed up for a road trip wearing a tuxedo."

Another big influence on me during my years at DePauw was former NBC correspondent Ken Bode. DePauw had just launched a brand-new, state-of-the-art media center, and Ken headed up the whole thing. The more time I spent around the newsroom, cameras, microphones, editing bays, and Ken, the more I started to focus and set my sights on what I needed to do to become a professional broadcast journalist. Ken became a great friend and mentor to me during those years, and his course on presidential politics inspired me to step it up in the classroom.

During my junior year at DePauw I traveled to the nation's capital as part of a Washington semester program based at American University. Along with taking classes at American, I got my first real taste of big-time news reporting when I landed an internship at CNN working directly with veteran news anchor Bernard Shaw. Being around Bernie was a truly amazing experience. This was after Saddam Hussein invaded Kuwait and the United States was in the run-up to Operation Desert Storm. Washington was electric with activity, and I was thrilled to be in the middle of all the excitement.

There were wall-to-wall news conferences and tons of congressional hearings about Iraq that CNN sent the other interns to. Perhaps to ensure I was plugged in ex-

actly where my gifts and talents could best be utilized, my particular job was to supply Bernie with popcorn during commercial breaks. I have no idea why this veteran broadcaster enjoyed munching on popcorn in between delivering the news, but he did, and my job was to keep the anchor happy. I always thought it was a strange snack for a television anchor since popcorn can easily stick to your teeth. But Bernie really liked his popcorn.

Another one of my important culinary jobs at CNN was to feed scripts into the teleprompter so Bernie could look straight ahead at the camera while reading the news. Teleprompter duty is pretty standard stuff for those getting their feet wet in television. Although there are always things that can go wrong, prompter work these days is much simpler than it was then because news scripts written on a standard computer can be electronically sent directly to the teleprompter screen. It's no longer necessary to print out pages and feed them into a machine.

But working for Bernie in 1990 with 1990 technology, my job was to take script pages and place them in sequence on a sort of conveyor belt that moved along at whatever speed fit the anchor's speaking style. One day during the lead-up to the Persian Gulf War, while Bernie was on the air live, I inadvertently knocked the switch to the fastest setting possible. Suddenly, script pages started flying around the CNN newsroom like an EF5 Kansas twister. It was a real mess.

Bernie deftly ad-libbed until a commercial break, when we could get things, not to mention script pages, sorted out. Mortified and sprawled on the studio floor scraping pages together, I heard that well-known, au-

thoritative Bernard Shaw voice proclaim, "We'll be right back." But I had serious doubts I would be. I was convinced this would be my last day in the CNN newsroom. After we were safely into the commercial, I apologized profusely, fully expecting a tap on my shoulder from the show's producer informing me my shift had just ended—permanently.

To my surprise, there was no tap on the shoulder, and Bernie nonchalantly dismissed the entire episode by saying, "Don't worry about it, kid. Happens all the time." Bernie was not upset in the least. Or at least he was gracious enough not to mention it and possibly destroy the confidence of an overeager college student who aspired to sit in a similar anchor chair one day. It was a lesson in graciousness I would never forget.

A few months later, with scripts or teleprompters nowhere to be found, Bernie stood on the rooftop of the Hotel Al Rasheed in downtown Baghdad and reported live to the world on the first incoming missiles and bombs of the Persian Gulf War. I have often wondered if Bernie's popcorn needs were sufficiently taken care of in between bomb blasts that night in Baghdad.

During summers at DePauw I would travel south from Greencastle to Hilton Head Island, South Carolina, where I worked at WJWJ-TV based in Beaufort. The first year there I was a volunteer, with no pay or benefits. To be perfectly honest, the sensational golf courses scattered around Hilton Head more than made up for the fact I wasn't getting paid. I started out being a gopher and doing whatever I was asked to do, but over time the folks at WJWJ gave me more and more responsibilities. It wasn't long before they started trusting me to shoot interviews, edit tape, and help put

together news packages. Eventually, I wore them down and they let me produce my own stories and even appear on air.

South Carolina was a good fit for me, so after I graduated from DePauw I returned to Hilton Head and became what WJWJ called their Low Country bureau reporter. I liked to call myself the Low Country bureau chief, but in reality I was a one-man band: reporter, cameraman, sound engineer, editor, janitor, driver, and office manager all wrapped into one. The station's mother ship was in Beaufort, but I was on my own out on Hilton Head Island, about an hour's drive away. I came up with my own story ideas, wrote scripts, shot video, and edited everything down for the evening newscast produced out of Beaufort.

There were all the normal go-it-alone TV reporter challenges like trying to frame up a stand-up shot by guesstimating how tall I was next to a tree or lamppost, or adjusting the camera focus by using a pile of leaves on the ground where I would eventually stand. But the tricky part of the job was my tight deadline. Even though the evening newscast was at 6:00 p.m., my personal deadline was 3:00 p.m. because I had to finish my story, then race to the Hilton Head airport so I could load my clunky three-quarter-inch tapes onto an old prop plane that made a daily afternoon flight across the Port Royal Sound to Beaufort.

If I happened to miss my 3:00 p.m. deadline and that plane, I would have to drive to Beaufort, deliver my tapes by hand, then trek all the way back to Hilton Head, a real pain for someone who was trying to maintain an evening social schedule. So to get my tapes on that flight, I was often forced to do my best Dale

Earnhardt impersonation and haul that beat-up old two-toned red and blue boat of a WJWJ station wagon from the bureau to the Hilton Head Airport. More times than I care to admit, I drove directly onto the tarmac of that little airport, hazard lights flashing, while I leaned on the horn the entire way to prevent the pilot from taking off without my tapes.

I've often thought the pilot of that prop plane probably got a big kick out of messing with the TV boy by intentionally idling at the end of the runway till he saw that red and blue blur of a station wagon careening down that dusty airport road, all so he could enjoy a nice Low Country belly laugh at my expense.

When I wasn't driving on the tarmac of the Hilton Head Airport you might find me lobbying my bosses about yet another golf course we needed to inform our viewers about. But more often than not, I would probably be on the beach shooting video for a piece about the nesting habits of the loggerhead sea turtle, or possibly at a town council meeting covering the latest raging Hilton Head political controversy. The annual debate over the color of the azaleas to be planted on the median of highway 278 was always particularly heated and scintillating.

I didn't earn much money in those days, so when I wasn't chasing down loggerhead turtles on the beach or thinking deep thoughts about the various shades of azaleas, I worked a few other jobs to help make ends meet. On the weekends I tended bar and waited tables at the local Applebee's. On weeknights, I delivered food all over the island for a company called Restaurants on the Go. Once I showed up at a home with a food order and a middle-aged man answered the door.

"Hey, you're the guy on channel six, right? I just saw you!" he said.

"Yessir," I replied. "Thanks for watching! Now, did you have the calzone or the crab legs?"

One big upside to working in South Carolina at the time was its rich history of political figures, not least of whom were the two sitting United States senators who would occasionally pass through Hilton Head for a fund-raiser or ribbon-cutting event of one kind or another.

Senator Fritz Hollings was a complete piece of southern construction with a deep drawl and laugh that was instantly identifiable in a crowded room. Hollings looked the part of a southern senator, with his silvery mane of hair and straight-from-central-casting looks. In fact, when Hollywood was looking to cast the role of a distinctive southern senator for a big scene in the Al Pacino film *City Hall*, Hollings was selected to play the part.

A former presidential contender during the 1984 Democratic primaries, Hollings had a bit of ignominious fame by being the third, and often forgotten, name on the once-heralded Gramm-Rudman-Hollings budget-balancing bill of 1985. Hollings, who always had spectacular navigational skills around the English language, said of his own balanced-budget legislation, "Gramm-Rudman-Hollings is a *baaad idea*—whose time has come."

Republican Senator Strom Thurmond, whose first campaign slogan exhorted voters to "Give a Young Man a Chance," was still a relatively young man of ninety-two when I was working in Hilton Head. I could never get out of my head the idea that Ol' Strom, as he was affec-

tionately known in South Carolina, was born the year the Wright brothers were still gliding. Strom had lived the entire history of American aviation and even jumped out of a few planes over Europe as a paratrooper during World War II.

On one particular occasion in the fancy ballroom of a Hilton Head hotel, both Fritz and Strom were working the room at the same time, always a treat. There was a sumptuous buffet table loaded with all sorts of Low Country offerings such as cucumber sandwiches, fried oysters, Frogmore stew, and what appeared to be a small mountain of fresh shrimp. Upon seeing this spectacular gastronomic presentation, Ol' Strom headed right for Shrimp Mountain and proclaimed, "Shrimp! I love shrimp!"

All perfectly fine and a totally understandable tribute given all the wonderful delicacies being displayed, but what followed next is something I will never forget. Not only did Strom unceremoniously start stuffing shrimp into his mouth, he also proceeded to stick handfuls of the catch directly into his pockets. No embarrassment. No napkins. No nothing. Just suit pockets filled with finely prepared fresh shrimp.

I thought, "Gheesh! Here's a long-standing United States senator, for gosh sakes. Can't his staff do a better job of getting this guy some shrimp once in a while?"

I guess Ol' Strom just wanted a little snack for the long car ride home.

A bemused smile on his face, Hollings took in the Strom buffet line episode as if he had watched this scene play out a thousand times before. I suppose we should all be thankful Strom didn't have a taste for cocktail sauce. Even though I was on a very strict budget in those days,

I am proud to report I did not stuff anything in my pockets for my own car ride home.

Not necessarily because I was an eyewitness to the Strom shrimp episode, but about this same time I started getting itchy and thinking it just might be time for me to move on. Hilton Head had been a fantastic learning experience for me, and the folks at WJWJ could not have been any nicer. But, counting my college summers, I had been working down there four years. You can do only so many loggerhead sea turtle nesting stories in one lifetime.

I think I actually made my decision to leave Hilton Head in the middle of a five-hour, knock-down, drag-out town council debate on whether the awnings at the local TGIF restaurant should be red and white, or, because of the sensibilities and sensitivities of a higher-end leisure town like Hilton Head, might the community be better served by the colors maroon and gray.

Before Fox News ever came along, my reporting on the Hilton Head TGIF color-scheme controversy was always "fair and balanced." But truth be told, I was a bit of a traditionalist and personally preferred red and white. I sure hope they got that color scheme figured out down there. To this day, I cannot pass up reading a good article about loggerhead sea turtles. And I definitely cannot walk by a buffet table with shrimp without breaking into a big Low Country grin.

Leaving Hilton Head with no specific job prospects, I decided to move back to Washington, D.C., a city that made a huge impression on me during my American University–Bernie Shaw days. My long-term goal was to work in Washington for one of the networks, so D.C. seemed like the perfect place for me to shake the sand

out of my sandals, regroup, get my résumé reel in order, and start sending out tapes. A few friends of mine had moved to Washington to attend law school and were living in a great house on Capitol Hill right behind the Supreme Court. Despite the rigors of studying law, my friends all seemed to be having a lot of fun. They also happened to have a spare bedroom, so that pretty much sealed the deal for me.

During the summer of 1994, about the same time Newt Gingrich and his band of Republican revolutionaries were on their way to winning the House of Representatives for the first time in forty years, I found myself living in D.C. and tending bar at the top of the Center Cafe in Washington's Union Station to make ends meet. I used every cent of my tip money for postage so I could send résumé tapes out across the country.

Although I knew I wasn't yet experienced enough to land a big-time reporting job in the D.C. television market, I made a few brassy attempts anyway, only to be shown the door. But thanks to the tip money from mixing margaritas at the Center Cafe, my tapes eventually stirred some interest in several local television markets across the country.

The next thing I knew, I was on the road to Rockford, Illinois, and a reporting job at WREX-TV. I briefly considered taking a job in Amarillo, Texas, but to an East Coast boy, Amarillo seemed to be about thirty-seven hours from the next closest town. No offense to the fine folks of Amarillo, but when I traveled there for an interview, I actually saw an honest-to-goodness tumbling tumbleweed, and it scared the daylights out of me. Just two hours from Chicago, Rockford seemed to have

its tumbleweed situation under control, so that choice was fairly easy.

Rockford was an interesting place to work. Although they seemed a little disinterested in the challenges facing the loggerhead, I worked on a wide range of other stories, including many dealing with crime, racism in schools, and drugs. I lived in downtown Rockford and once produced a piece about drug dealers in my own neighborhood by setting up the camera in my apartment and shooting the story out my kitchen window: the offer of drugs, exchange of cash, arrival of the police, everything. If I hadn't had to go into the station to edit my piece, I could have stayed in my pajamas all day and finished the story sitting at my kitchen table while drinking a cup of coffee.

After Rockford, I headed south to North Carolina where I took a job as a general assignment reporter at the highly rated CBS affiliate in Raleigh, WRAL-TV. Over the course of my career in journalism, I've had a lot of interesting first days on the job, but my first twenty-four hours at WRAL took the cake.

The day started out tame enough, with my photographer and me heading to the University of North Carolina in Chapel Hill to produce a story about Title IX college sports programs. While we were on the UNC campus getting ready to do some on-camera interviews we got a call on the radio that a tornado was about to touch down near Zebulon, a very small town about twenty miles east of Raleigh.

Unceremoniously, we threw all our equipment into the van and raced toward Zebulon, about an hour's drive from Chapel Hill. While we were on the road approaching the town we looked out our van window and saw a

funnel cloud. We stopped along the road so the photographer could shoot video of the tornado touching down, then we continued to a trailer park where several dozen homes had been damaged or destroyed.

It was a mess, a heartbreaking disaster area with several folks milling around, confused, crying, and trying to reconnect with their loved ones. I remember trying to help a woman find her young daughter when suddenly a police officer came by and hollered, "There's another one coming. Another one is coming. Another one is coming!"

All of a sudden everyone started running in the same direction toward a ditch by the side of the road. Being in the TV business, we, of course, shot video up until the last second before we, too, dove into the ditch and hunkered down for dear life with everyone else. Thankfully, the second funnel cloud kept moving and touched down about a mile away from where we were.

Eventually my cameraman and I shot some more video, and with as much sensitivity as we could conducted interviews with several local folks, some of whom had lost everything. Despite the loss of property, everyone, including me, was extremely thankful there was no loss of life.

Meanwhile, the station sent a transmission truck to meet up with us so we could do live reports from the scene. I wound up doing live shots all night long and producing a full package for WRAL's 11:00 p.m. newscast. In the middle of gathering the elements needed for my story, I was also doing live hits throughout the evening for various CBS affiliates across the country.

Barely making it back to my apartment in Raleigh for a few hours' sleep, I returned to Zebulon at first light for

appearances on the CBS morning show and some live walk-and-talks to show the path of the storm and the devastation. I had only been in Raleigh for a few days and was still living out of a suitcase. I barely knew the names of the anchors back at the station, let alone my fellow reporters. I was so new to the area I had to ask folks around me for the correct pronunciation of Zebulon seconds before I went on the air for the first time. I had pretty much been on the air nonstop for the better part of twenty-four hours, all on my first day on the job.

The following day, cameraman Mark Copeland and I went to the nearby town of Lizard Lick about five miles west of Zebulon to do some storm aftermath stories. Lizard Lick didn't even have a stoplight in 1996 and was basically just a crossroads on the map with a small diner and gas station. When Mark and I walked into the diner, six big-bellied regulars were at the counter eating breakfast. As I walked through the screen door all six of those burly guys turned to me and said, "Well, hiyaah, Bret!" like they had known me their entire lives.

With all the affiliate reporting I had been doing—and this just my second day on the job—I had probably appeared on WRAL only three or four times over the past twelve hours, and these guys at this small diner in the middle of nowhere were calling me by my first name. That encounter convinced me not only how popular WRAL was throughout the region, but it was a good reminder of the vital, up-close, on-the-ground role local reporters can play in a community, whether they are diving into the same ditch with their viewers or not.

Many memories from those early days filled my mind as I cruised along I-85 and edged my way over to the right lane for the Georgia Tech exit and the final few

blocks to the Fox bureau. A great space in the Georgia Public Television complex, the bureau was a huge step up from just a few years before when the entirety of the Atlanta bureau was in the living room of my 600-square-foot apartment.

I absolutely loved working at WRAL and living in Raleigh, but when the brand-new Fox News Channel came along and offered me a chance to open a regional bureau in my hometown of Atlanta, I thought I had died and gone to heaven.

The only resources I had during those early days in Atlanta were a clunky fax machine, a cell phone about the size of a loaf of bread, and an end-of-the-world supply of Pizza Combos and Diet Coke. This was early 1998, about the same time news headlines across the country were screaming with stories about President Clinton and his relationship with former White House intern Monica Lewinsky. While the impeachment drums were beating on Capitol Hill and special prosecutor Ken Starr was becoming a household name, I busied myself with covering any number of non-Monica stories across the southeast—and there were plenty.

In a few short years our fledgling Atlanta bureau had grown into a fully functioning news operation with full-time camera operators, producers, and even some real office space. My bosses in New York also hired a full-time bureau chief named Sharon Fain so I could work on stories 100 percent of the time and not have to worry about the million and one logistical details a bureau chief needs to deal with.

It wasn't long before the Atlanta bureau earned the reputation within Fox for being the crazy folks who would go anywhere, at any moment, to cover stories

that no one else wanted or were too busy to cover: tornadoes, hurricanes, the search for the Olympic Park bomber in the North Carolina mountains, Timothy McVeigh, and the Elián González story that took me to Cuba several times, just to name a few.

We also did our fair share of water-cooler/refrigerator-magnet stories, such as lawnmower racing in Alabama, UFO sightings in North Carolina, and the population explosion of rodents called nutria in Louisiana. Nutria became such a problem the state actually encouraged restaurants to come up with nutria dishes for their menus.

I was easily spending three weeks out of each month on the road in those days. I was traveling so much I sometimes wondered why I kept an apartment at all. Maybe I should have just bought a cot and slept in the bureau like those congressmen who sleep in their Capitol Hill offices. Given the fact that most of my colleagues had actually seen my apartment and knew where neatness ranked on my personal hierarchy of needs pyramid, I doubt they would have gone along with that idea for very long.

I was on the road for such long stretches I am fairly certain I still hold some Guinness Book records for killing the most apartment plants in a year. It wasn't just me. Everyone in the Atlanta bureau had the same pick up and go mentality. In fact, it was a bureau requirement that we all have go-bags stuffed with fresh clothes and toiletries so we could pick up and roll on a moment's notice.

When it came to catching last-minute flights to the next news hot spot, we had it down to an absolute science. Upon receiving word we were needed somewhere

across the southeast to cover a story, several of us would immediately pile into a car or a van loaded with all our television equipment and race to Atlanta's Hartsfield Airport. Pulling up to the outside drop-off point, our cameraperson would jump out to find the special baggage handlers we generously tipped to move our cases of equipment onto the plane. My producer Malinda Adams or I would run to the counter to buy tickets while the other would park the car. We would typically reassemble at the gate and all bundle onto our plane to wherever just as the doors were about to close.

It was a matter of bureau pride with us. If the bosses in New York or Washington called to see if we could travel that day to report a story, we responded yes even before we knew where we were going. I was convinced that if they ever held any kind of news bureau Olympics and the event was covering spot news, my colleagues in the Fox Atlanta bureau would have been gold-medal winners. Sometimes this life was glamorous, but mostly it was just a lot of endless sixteen-hour days, and I often wondered how someone with a family could ever handle such a hectic schedule. Those rare, reflective moments didn't last very long, however, because it was always time to head off to the next hot spot.

Despite the fact that I loved being based in Atlanta and had a wide range of stories to choose from, after covering fifteen hurricanes and tropical storms for the network, I sometimes worried I was being typecast as Hurricane Guy and perhaps undermining my chances to be assigned to the political stories I loved doing.

Don't get me wrong. Hurricanes, tropical storms, and tornadoes are huge stories that need to be covered and

covered well. Folks across the country are very interested in extreme weather events, and those living in the path of destruction certainly deserve to have their stories told. But with my previous stints in Washington and my keen interest in political news, while handling all my other story assignments I was constantly lobbying the network bosses to let me produce political pieces every chance I got.

Fox had been extremely fortunate to recruit longtime ABC News White House Correspondent Brit Hume to the network, and he and his team in Washington had launched an incredibly interesting political news show called *Special Report* that was really starting to catch on. Whenever I wasn't tracking hurricanes or doing manhunt stories in the mountains of North Carolina, I was constantly looking for creative ways to get southern political stories into the mix, and specifically onto Brit's show.

Over time, the folks in Washington and New York took notice of my pieces, often southern-fried and spiced with a healthy dose of local color. Brit was incredibly supportive and encouraged me to do as much as I could without shirking the normal news responsibilities expected out of a regional bureau.

Life was good. The Atlanta bureau was humming. I was being encouraged to produce more stories about southern politics, and at a moment's notice I was parachuting into one exciting story after another. I was definitely a young man in a hurry and living the lifestyle where one late-night phone call could send me to the airport and three weeks on the road without a break. That is exactly what happened in November of 2000 when the network sent me to Nashville to cover the Al

Gore victory—or defeat—story, depending on Election Day results.

I packed relatively light for Nashville, fully expecting it to be two days at most, win or lose. But after election night produced no clear winner, I was told to head to the center of the storm, which seemed to be the Panhandle of Florida. After a day in the Panhandle, and still relying on my two-day clothes supply as if I were tracking the uncertain path of a raging hurricane, I was instructed to divert to Tallahassee where the front lines of the Bush–Gore legal battle were taking shape.

With my interest in politics and having covered all those hurricanes and tornadoes for the network, I felt right at home in Tallahassee, working, arguably, in the middle of the nation's largest political storm of the past hundred years. I had the great fortune of being able to work the Florida recount story with veteran reporter Jim Angle. For a month Jim and I worked side by side in the back of a U-Haul truck we rented and parked right outside the courthouse in Tallahassee. Working in extremely tight quarters, Jim and I were forced to become instant friends, not to mention instant experts on any number of election topics, including a new one on me called a voting card chad.

Jim and I soon realized that not only did we have to become experts on your everyday run-of-the-mill chads, there was an evolving bit of expertise to be had in dented chads, dimpled chads, perforated chads, and something that seemed to be driving folks crazy down in Palm Beach County called butterfly ballots. Throw in all the nuances and ambiguities of Florida election law, and the expectation that we be able to wake up at 3:00 a.m. and clearly articulate the differences between

Volusia, Broward, Palm Beach, Miami Dade, and Nassau counties, and you get an idea what we and everyone else covering that monster of a story were up against.

The Bush-Gore recount was unlike any story I had ever covered. Typically news divisions will have a morning meeting to map out the day's coverage, but with the Florida recount, by the time that first idea emanated from the morning meeting, the story on the ground had already changed at least three times. We had to constantly be on our toes to make sure we didn't miss the latest developments that could erupt at a moment's notice and in any one of Florida's sixty-seven counties.

With the American presidency hanging in the balance, it didn't get any bigger than the Florida recount. But despite all the pressure associated with covering such a historic moment in American politics, I was having the time of my life. After the Florida recount, I definitely had the bug to do political reporting full time, and that probably meant having to travel directly into the well-formed eye of just about every major political storm out there—Washington, D.C.

As I drove past Atlanta's iconic Varsity restaurant on this brilliant September morning—still holding out hope for that always elusive postwork bucket of balls—I wondered what the bosses in Washington or New York might be wanting from me today.

As was my habit driving to the bureau, I scanned the radio dial to see if there was any buzz about anything, and I quickly picked up on a story about a plane that hit an office building in New York City. Parking in my normal space outside the bureau, I started to think that if a building in Manhattan had accidently been hit by

a plane, the New York folks would probably have their hands full for the morning, leaving me to come up with my own story for the day.

Fine with me. I always had about forty-three different political stories rolling around in my head and ready to pitch at a moment's notice, all part of my master plan to get on Brit's show as often as possible and reinforce my case for working in Washington full time.

As I walked into the Fox Atlanta bureau on the morning of September 11, 2001, I had no idea that within fifteen minutes I would be racing out the same door with my producer Joe Hirsch on our way to Washington, D.C., two-day go-bag slung over my shoulder. How could I possibly know this would be a one-way trip and my last day working in Atlanta?

CHAPTER TWO

Together as One

My first few weeks in Washington were an absolute blur. With nearly three thousand dead at the hands of terrorists, it was extremely difficult to process all that had taken place, let alone get a fix on what the future might hold.

When I first arrived in Washington on the evening of September 11, the Pentagon was in flames and rescue teams were still searching for survivors. Smelling the acrid smoke, seeing the flames, and looking down on the gruesome scene of that crushed outer ring, all within my first five minutes in Washington, affected me deeply. The dead at the Pentagon and the World Trade Center and the passengers and crews on those four airliners were fellow Americans. We were all attacked on that horrific day, and I had been given the job of reporting on the people who were responsible for it and those planning on doing something about it.

Starting very early on the morning of September 12, I went to the Pentagon every day to do live shots for

Fox affiliates across the country. Producing taped news packages, live stand-ups, and what are called talk-backs with local anchors in various markets, I stood in front of the still smoldering Pentagon and talked with Jim, Sally, Jen, Alex, Bob, and Kathy in St. Louis, Atlanta, Detroit, L.A., Miami, Honolulu, and just about everywhere in between.

Apart from the tragedy, trauma, and emotion I shared with my countrymen, from a purely journalistic stand-point, I simply didn't want to screw it up. The American people had taken a serious hit, and I was humbled to be one of many journalists who went to work during those days with a renewed sobriety about the importance of what we did.

As tragedy often does, the attacks brought the American people and the politicians in Washington together as I had never seen before. I will never forget the images of those members of Congress—Republicans, Democrats, and Independents—descending the east steps of the United States Capitol the evening of September 11 and singing "God Bless America."

After I had reported for a few weeks outside the Pentagon, my bosses at Fox decided to send me inside the building to cover the Department of Defense, the emerging military campaign to root out the Taliban and al Qaeda in Afghanistan, and the manhunt for Usama bin Laden (UBL—the official government designation for al Qaeda's #1 terrorist). With all branches of the U.S. military based at the Pentagon and its seventeen-plus miles of corridors and thousands of offices, I have to admit I was more than a bit confused about the best way to go about covering the place.

The long-timers at the Pentagon had given it the

not-so-affectionate nickname the Puzzle Palace. Fair enough. But my preferred phrase for reporting the news there was "news by quilt." You would get one piece of the quilt over at the Marines and another at the Army; then more pieces from the Air Force and Navy. Soon, after making your morning rounds talking to defense officials and military commanders scattered throughout the building, you would return to the media work space and assemble the pieces collected throughout the day. If you were lucky, you could stitch together, piece by piece, a whole quilt of a story that made a little more sense than the individual pieces sometimes did.

One of the most colorful pieces of that vast Pentagon quilt, of course, was none other than the secretary of defense himself, Donald Rumsfeld. During the early days of the war in Afghanistan and later, during the invasion of Iraq, Secretary Rumsfeld's afternoon Q&A sessions with reporters became must-see TV. To those following developments in Washington closely during those days, the Pentagon briefing room became as familiar as their own living rooms.

Secretary Rumsfeld could handle a question better than just about any public figure I'd ever come across. Let me rephrase that: Secretary Rumsfeld could *not* answer a question better than just about any public figure I'd ever come across. He was so adept at controlling the information flow from his command post at the podium that soon everyone started referring to his non-answer answers as Rummyspeak.

If you could summon the courage to engage Rumsfeld on a particular topic you better be solid, not only on the basic premise of your question but also on any information or presuppositions you stuck

in before you ever got to your question. If you violated those rules, got sloppy, or didn't have your reportorial act together in some other way, more times than not Rumsfeld would turn the whole thing around on you before a nationwide live television audience.

During one of those briefings, Rumsfeld turned the tables on one hapless reporter by saying,

"You're beginning with an illogical premise and proceeding perfectly logically to an illogical conclusion, which is a dangerous thing to do."

Washington journalists are never very high on the nation's Most Adorable list. With the distinct possibility of witnessing a totally eviscerated reporter left mumbling to himself and gasping for air, those news conferences soon rocketed Rummy, as he became known, to what many considered to be rock-star status—at least by Washington public policy standards.

That daily, high-stakes, high-wire briefing room atmosphere, with the good chance of seeing a reporter completely Rummified live and nationwide, soon made those sessions popular television fare, and not just to devotees of C-SPAN. The briefings sometimes surpassed the popular soaps *Days of our Lives* and *As the World Turns* in the daytime television ratings. As a result, reporters covering the Pentagon in those days felt intense pressure to deliver a coherent question and come across as halfway respectable.

Once, one of my esteemed Pentagon colleagues, Jim Miklaszewski of NBC, tried to press Rumsfeld on evidence that did or did not link Saddam Hussein to al Qaeda. The exchange launched a quote that went round the world:

Jim Miklaszewski: There are reports that there is no evidence of a direct link between Baghdad and some of these terrorist organizations.

Secretary Rumsfeld: There are known knowns; there are things we know we know. We also know there are known unknowns; that is to say, we know there are some things that we know we do not know. But there are also unknown unknowns; the ones we don't know we don't know.

Jim, ever the quintessential and fearless pro, boldly dove back in to attempt a redemptive follow-up. Playing along with the rules of Rummyspeak, he proceeded to ask the secretary if the answer to his particular question might be found in the "unknown unknown" category. Rumsfeld, employing the tools of any self-respecting rock star, simply refused to answer.

Like most of my Pentagon colleagues, I mixed it up many times with Secretary Rumsfeld during my years there. A common line of questioning during my early days dealt with the whereabouts of Usama bin Laden: "Do you know where he is? Do you have a track on him? Are you close to catching him? Where was the last 'known known' place he was seen?"

Rumsfeld's answers to me were always the same—always colorful, but never of much true news value: "It's like running around the barnyard chasing a chicken. Until you get it [the chicken], you don't have it."

Although my first question at news conferences was typically on the news of the day, more times than not my follow-up would always be a variation of the "Where is UBL?" question. I asked the UBL question so many

times, the second I started to segue to my follow-up I would hear groans from several of my briefing room colleagues.

Once, in 2002, when we were traveling with Rumsfeld to Afghanistan, about three hours into the flight one of his aides came back to where the reporters were to tell us the secretary would like to have a press availability. Dutifully, we grabbed our notebooks and recorders and made our way to the front of the plane where Rumsfeld was sitting behind a desk in his very cramped office.

After a brief statement about the purpose of the trip, Secretary Rumsfeld opened it up for questions. Associated Press reporter Bob Burns, a fantastic guy and great reporter, asked about Pakistan and whether that nation was playing both sides of the street in efforts to track down bin Laden and other members of al Qaeda. Rumsfeld answered with one of his classic nonanswer award winners, and then he turned to me.

I could sense all those crammed-in reporters collectively cringe, knowing that even flying across the Atlantic my "Where is bin Laden?" question was about to be unfurled. I figured if I couldn't extract any decent answers at sea level, perhaps 35,000 feet up might do the trick. But sensing a wave of familiarity washing over my colleagues, I decided to switch it up a little. "Mr. Secretary," I asked, "do you think Usama bin Laden knows where you are right now?"

Not only did Rumsfeld start laughing, all the reporters did, too. I think I cleared a major hurdle that day with all those veteran defense reporters. From that day forward whenever I asked my Usama question the mumbles and groans never rose above a certain decibel level.

During the remainder of 2002 I made several trips

to Afghanistan and saw firsthand some amazing scenes. Once, traveling with Chairman of the Joint Chiefs of Staff General Richard Myers, we visited a rural area a few hours outside Kabul where an army unit was helping a small village get back on its feet after years of Taliban rule. A school for boys *and girls* was being constructed. A water system was going in. Farmers were being helped with several agricultural projects. On and on.

To my surprise, the man who seemed to be in charge was a young American Army captain. From the way the villagers approached him with problems and the way they responded when he spoke, if I didn't know any better I would say he was the unofficial town mayor. He didn't speak their language very well, but somehow he was able to communicate with them just fine. With his sunny disposition and calm demeanor, you could see he was having a huge impact on this dusty corner of the world.

As I got a bit nearer and saw this soldier up close and interacting with the villagers, I was amazed to see he was a Midwestern boy in his twenties. He looked like he was sixteen years old and barely shaving. And he was running this entire town. Truly an amazing sight; it was pure, from-the-gut, on-the-ground, inspirational leadership at its best, and totally impressive to observe. From my vantage point that Soldier-Mayor-Midwest *Kid* had everything it took to run just about any company or represent any congressional district in America.

That was just one of many scenes I witnessed of young soldiers who were making a huge difference in the lives of people in Afghanistan. That episode made me double down in my efforts to tell as many of their on-the-ground stories as I possibly could.

To be sure, there are always mistakes, mishaps, and even horrible decisions made by military and civilian leaders during wartime, and I covered plenty of those as well. But I made a special point to keep an eye out for those young soldiers, men and women from all over America, who were making a real difference in the lives of people halfway around the world and representing us in extremely difficult circumstances.

When I first arrived in Washington in September 2001, I had no idea my move was going to be permanent. My first few weeks in D.C. I lived in a Holiday Inn just a block from the Fox bureau, not far from the U.S. Capitol. After a few weeks it seemed like the folks in the Washington bureau wanted me to stick around; at least no one told me to go back home to Atlanta.

Still relying on the small go-bag of clothes I left Atlanta with, I found the closest Brooks Brothers and did a thirty-minute power shop to buy clothes to hold me over. There was so much going on in Washington I never even had time to return to Atlanta to get my things. Fox was nice enough to hire movers to go to my apartment, gather up my stuff, load it all on a truck, and bring it to me in Washington. My longtime friend Dave Tafuri found me a small apartment on Calvert Street in the Adams Morgan neighborhood of the city. Dave lived on the third floor of the same building, while my place was a small one-bedroom unit on the first floor.

When my boxes from Atlanta finally arrived, the movers piled them in the center of the living room of the small place on Calvert Street I was now calling home. One weekend, when I had a few hours to catch my breath, I started to unpack the boxes. Two boxes in I discovered the movers had neatly wrapped all my dishes.

Very nice of them. The only problem: the dishes were all caked with food, just the way I'd left them in my sink when I left Atlanta a month earlier.

Unwrapping those dishes was like working at an archaeological dig at Pompeii. I had this bizarre vision of a bespectacled archaeologist clutching his dusting brush in one hand and magnifying glass in the other as he performed a squinty-eyed examination and documented in his journal all the ridges and gradations of a month-old half-eaten pizza combo. These movers were really conscientious about their work. Each dirty fork, grimy plate, and cruddy cup was individually wrapped in tissue paper like a Christmas gift from Tiffany.

After a few more exciting archaeological finds, I started to break into a cold sweat. I still had not come across the one item I absolutely needed for survival. Finally, as I opened up the last box, I let out a giant exhale. My Titleist AP2 irons and TaylorMade Tour Burner woods had successfully made the trip north. I now had everything I needed to survive not only in D.C. but also on the seventeenth fairway at Congressional Country Club—like I would ever get a chance to play there!

In between going to the Pentagon every day and making trips to Afghanistan, I tried my best to piece together as much of a social life as I could during my first year in Washington. My social life was a puzzle palace unto itself, with several friends trying their best to provide some of the missing pieces.

Dave Tafuri, an associate at a big D.C. law firm, knew the crazy hours I was working at the Pentagon and how much I was traveling overseas. Dave worked long hours, too, but he never seemed to have a problem filling his evenings with one spectacular date after another. Feel-

ing a bit merciful toward me, he took it upon himself to introduce me to some young ladies who wouldn't be thrown by my work and travel schedule. But for all his good intentions, Dave was striking out. After a series of particularly painful blind dates, I told Dave, "No more." And I meant it. I think I would have actually volunteered for extra trips into the war zone to avoid hearing one more of Dave's "Dude, she's hot. It'll be fun!"

Before long, matchmaker Dave had one more special project up his sleeve. Just to get him off my back, I said yes to one final blind date he and the girl he was dating at the time, Kathryn Minor, decided would be a perfect match for me. I'd heard that "perfect match" language before, so it was with some reluctance that I went along with their plan. I agreed to go with Dave, Kathryn, and "this girl from Chicago" to a Rolling Stones concert at FedEx Field in the Maryland suburbs just outside D.C. I knew the Stones would have it cranked all the way up to eleven, so if this turned out to be like any of Dave's other picks of the week, at least Keith Richards's guitar licks would be loud enough to fill those torturous blind-date moments of silence.

On the night of October 4, 2002, we decided to meet at a place called the Firefly in D.C. before we drove together to the concert in Dave's Defender. Dave and I pulled up a few minutes late and walked into the Firefly to scan the crowd. Sitting at a table in the corner, I saw Kathryn and a very attractive brunette—the girl from Chicago, Amy Hills. I knew it didn't guarantee we would have a fun night, but I could already see that Amy from Chicago was not only gorgeous but also had this incredible smile. More than a little relieved, I turned to matchmaker-in-chief Tafuri and said, "Way to go, Dave!"

From the moment I walked into Firefly and sat down at her table, Amy and I started talking, laughing, and bantering. Amy is a very grounded Midwestern girl who went to Southern Methodist University in Dallas with Kathryn. She'd also spent time working in New York City, so nothing about Washington intimidated her—least of all me.

The bantering and kibitzing continued through our ride to FedEx Field, into the stadium, finding our seats, during the concert, and didn't stop till we parted company about 1:00 a.m. after we all got back to D.C. Amy had told her parents she was going to Washington for the weekend and would be meeting this guy who was on television. Her very wise and protective father replied, "Everybody in D.C. says they are on television." We laughed about that and every other topic that came up over the weekend as we did some sightseeing and hit several restaurants and clubs around town.

For me, it was a Hollywood romance whirlwind weekend, and I had the time of my life. Safe to say, I was totally smitten, completely head over heels for Amy within the first five minutes of talking to her. In fact, in my head the Checklist was completely marked up:

Very attractive/hot—*Check.*
Funny/blast to talk to—*Check.*
Confident—*Check.*
Interesting—*Check.*
Puts me in my place when required—*Check.*
Did I say hot already? *Check. Check. Check.*

Despite my obvious interest in Amy and the great time we had together all weekend, I was having an ex-

tremely difficult time reading her interest level, if any, in me. The weekend came to an end, and on Sunday afternoon Kathryn and I drove Amy to Reagan National so she could catch her flight back home to Chicago where she worked for the Eli Lilly pharmaceutical company. After a hug, a small kiss good-bye, and promises to stay in touch, I hopped back into the car. With no hesitation or pretense, I turned to Kathryn and said something I had never said to anyone or about anyone.

"I am going to marry that girl."

Over the next several weeks, Amy and I spent a lot of time on the phone together. I even made a few surprise trips to see her in Chicago. Eventually, I was able to convince Amy to come to D.C. to visit me. So a few weeks later, after returning from yet another trip to Afghanistan, I prepared for a historic trip of another kind—Amy Hills to Washington. Unfortunately, I wouldn't have the Rolling Stones as my backup band this time around. But after all those phone conversations, Amy knew she had a complete puppy dog on her hands who was madly in love with her.

There were still a few problems with the relationship, however. I was not altogether sure Amy was into me as much as I was into her. The other problem had to do with our completely different worldviews on the highly controversial topic of neatness. The first time I visited Amy's condo in Chicago, I knew instantly I was in the presence of a world-class, gold-medal neat freak. Amy was probably the most organized person I had ever met. Every piece of clothing she owned, every towel, every sheet was perfectly folded and in its proper place. I think she might have coined the phrase "a thing for every place—and a place for every thing."

I think I had that motto monogrammed somewhere, but it must have gotten buried under the ten tons of other stuff I had filed throughout my apartment.

Just like my place in Atlanta, my Calvert Street apartment would have easily qualified as a FEMA debris removal area. The entire "doing laundry" fad was just not something that ever took with me. I, of course, was organized in other areas of my life, but with laundry—specifically dirty laundry—I had a mental block. I had a complete aversion to keeping my clothes clean, folded, put away, and all those other things some people—including Amy—seemed to find important. Someone looking in on my situation, and specifically my apartment, might have gotten the idea I had been traumatized by a rogue Maytag as a child. Whatever the reason, having dirty laundry lying around, in the grand scheme of things, simply never bothered me. It was just not something I really thought about—let alone cared about. Until now.

I so desperately wanted to impress my completely adorable neat freak dream girl from Chicago, I knew I better make an effort to clean my place or else. If I didn't do something fast, Amy might get the impression I was one of those cliché unkempt bachelors who sits around till all hours of the morning in his boxer shorts, tripping over pizza boxes and trying to find the television clicker so he can catch the 2:00 a.m. ET repeat of *Sports Center*.

As I said, I certainly didn't want Amy to get that impression.

Having just returned from overseas, I had my normal Mount Vesuvius pile of dirty clothes accumulated after several days on the road. I immediately dumped the just-back-from-Afghanistan pile directly on top of the

already existing mountain in my apartment. Slight problem. By now, Amy had undoubtedly received some top-secret intelligence briefings from my double-agent friends who spilled the beans about my disinclination toward tidiness. I clearly got the idea that during her upcoming trip Amy wanted to conduct her own firsthand investigation of my place to get a better picture of how serious the situation was.

One day back from Afghanistan, and just twenty-four hours before Amy's visit, I was having a very busy day at the Pentagon: two separate briefings, four live shots for the network, and a full news package for Brit Hume's *Special Report*. With not much discretionary time on my schedule to make my place presentable, and with Amy arriving the next day, if I didn't get my act together, I would be toast.

When I finally got home that night, just hours before Amy's arrival, I had the brilliant idea I could save a ton of time washing and drying if I simply transferred all my dirty clothes to my car for the weekend. I could borrow another car while Amy was in town, and if I could just keep my own car out of sight, I should be home free.

After carrying seven loads of dirty clothes to my car out on Calvert Street, I had successfully dismantled Mount Vesuvius, shirt by dirty shirt. However, performing a last-minute quality control check, I realized there were still five or six armloads of dirty laundry scattered helter-skelter in various nooks and crannies throughout my apartment. The Silver Bullet, as my Mitsubishi Diamante was called, was already filled to the roof. And I was afraid if I tried to crack open the door to slip in just one more pair of boxers, my dirty laundry and I would

be sprawled all over Calvert Street and halfway down to the Washington Monument.

Being the get-it-done, achieve-the-objective kind of guy I am, I systematically laid out my options:

Number 1. I could throw out the remaining dirty clothes and take the financial loss.

Number 2. I could ask Dave to hide the clothes in one of his closets.

Number 3. I could simply bundle all the remaining dirty clothes into a big pile, place them along the back wall of my bedroom, and cover the whole thing up with two king-size black sheets. In short, create sort of an elongated bean-bag-chair-of-an-intergalactic-black-hole-inspired piece of bedroom-wall-furniture-art that wouldn't draw too much attention. With the lights down low and candles burning to deaden the smell, I was confident the large black mound would be as inconspicuous as any large black mound of dirty laundry possibly could be.

To pull this off, I would need to pick Amy up at the airport in another car, since the Silver Bullet would be pulling Maytag duty on Calvert Street. Dave, who definitely thought option number three was much better than number two, lent me his Defender for the weekend—the same car we'd used to go to the Rolling Stones concert back in October.

I would have to tell a bit of a white lie if Amy asked why I didn't have my own car. I was fairly certain it wasn't in the Bible, but I remembered something someone once said about "all's fair in love and war." And this was definitely about love—and specifically doing everything I possibly could to convince Amy I was the perfect "no-baggage-no-issues" guy for her.

Amy arrived at Reagan National Airport right on time, and I was out front waiting for her in Dave's Defender.

"Isn't this Dave's car?" she immediately asked after I greeted her with a big hug.

"Yes, mine is in the shop," I replied.

Trying to change the topic and put my sinful ways behind me, I thought my transgression wouldn't be as bad if I intimated that I'd borrowed Dave's car for sentimental reasons.

"It's hard to believe we talked right back there just two months ago driving to the Stones concert. Remember?"

Having taken great pains to not drive anywhere near the Silver Bullet, when we arrived at my place we went inside so I could give Amy the quick tour before dinner. With the lights down low, music playing, and candles burning, I have to admit, that little one-bedroom apartment had never looked so good—a serious bachelor pad of the first order. Feeling a little cocky about the way the place looked and smelled, I decided to go for it and give Amy the expanded tour and show her my bedroom. Immediately, Amy's eyes went straight to the big black invisible mound along the far wall.

"What is that?" Amy asked.

"What is what?" I replied.

"That big pile against the wall! Is there a dead body under there? Are those dirty clothes? Oh my gosh!" she exclaimed.

Like an astronomer discovering a brand-new galaxy, Amy rushed over to the black hole and immediately rolled back the sheets, exposing all the dirty clothes the Silver Bullet didn't have space for and Dave didn't have

the stomach for. I looked at Amy and smiled. "Sorry, I ran out of time," I said.

And, as if it really needed saying: "I was hoping you wouldn't see that."

I got the impression Amy was running numbers in her head as she performed a cost-benefit analysis to determine if her investment in the Bret Baier Project could possibly be worth the effort. By the look in her eyes, I could see that if this Baier-Hills merger was going to stay on track, I was going to need to step it up a few notches in the personal hygiene department. But on second thought, maybe this wasn't such a bad strategy after all. When you are totally outmatched and outclassed on every level by the one girl on the planet you are desperately in love with, go for the sympathy vote and try to get that "he'll never make it without me" vibe going.

Having barely survived Operation Dirty Laundry and now on our way out the door to go to dinner, Amy stopped to admire a picture I had on the wall.

"That's a great picture of you with your father," she said.

"Uh, Amy. That's not my father. That's Secretary of Defense Donald Rumsfeld," I replied.

I smiled and actually felt a little relieved. To be sure, I needed more than a little help in the area of neatness. But perhaps I would be able to help Amy in the area of politics and public affairs. Despite several complaints that someone in the neighborhood was living in their car, Amy never did get a chance to see the Silver Bullet before she left for Chicago. Now that would have been a real deal-killer.

Throughout this entire period I continued to travel to Chicago to see as much of Amy as possible. If I wasn't

traveling overseas, I would typically take off for Chicago right after work on Friday evening and return to D.C. on the earliest Monday morning flight I could catch. It was a horrible commute to say the least. But if I could get two full days with Amy, it was fine by me, so I guess you could say it was the best worst commute I ever had.

I was so into Amy, I discovered romantic bones in me I never knew I had.

Once, I called to wish her happy birthday, which Amy found very sweet. I told her to go to her door because I'd had a surprise gift sent to her. I stayed on the phone as she opened the door only to see me standing there with an armful of roses. It helped that I was on a first-name basis with the security guy in her building. A modest tip didn't hurt, either.

Now in total, unabashed, dogged pursuit, I was pulling out all the stops in my efforts to convince Amy I was the one. Knowing how incredibly close Amy was to her parents and her three brothers, including a twin, I decided to fight fire with fire. During the 2002 Christmas holidays, knowing she would be with her family in Naples, Florida, I decided to take my brother, Tim, and my mother on a Christmas vacation, too.

To Naples, Florida, of course.

Not only could I spend time with Amy, but I would be able to meet her parents for the first time. It was also an opportunity for me to introduce my mother and brother to Amy and her family. The trip to Florida was strictly about romance and getting the families together. The fact that Naples has several sensational golf courses was only a minor consideration.

Our first day there, before the great family-to-family meeting was scheduled to take place, my brother,

mother, and I went to a course called Tiburon to play a round of golf. The club pro informed us we were next up, but he said he needed to send us out with a fourth, someone we didn't know. All was fine for the first few holes. The gentleman playing with us was nice enough, but he was definitely not a great golfer. I could see this had the potential for being a very long round. After Tim and I hit our tee shots on the fourteenth hole, the stray player we picked up shanked his ball very badly, firing it directly toward my mother, who was standing by the golf cart just fifteen yards away. The ball hit my mom in the head, and she immediately started bleeding. This wasn't just a little amount of blood, either; this was MASH unit blood all over my mother's face, the towel I was holding on her head, and the cart. Blood was gushing everywhere.

Pedal to the metal on the golf cart, we trailed blood all the way from the fourteenth tee to the clubhouse, where we called 911 for an ambulance. Soon we found ourselves in the Naples Community Hospital emergency room.

Some pain medication and twenty-four stiches later, Mom was starting to feel a little better about things. In the meantime, hearing about the incident, Amy and her folks rushed to be with us in the emergency room. I eventually walked my mom out of the ER and into the waiting room where everyone was gathered. With bandages all over her head, my mother, of course, immediately apologized to Amy's folks for the way she looked.

Not exactly how I planned on meeting Amy's family for the first time, either, but there we were in the Naples Community Hospital ER making all the family intro-

ductions as if we were in the lobby of the Ritz-Carlton. Little did we know that before too much time had passed, both our families would be spending more time together in hospital waiting rooms than we could ever imagine.

The year 2003 was shaping up to be a huge news year in Washington, so I knew I was going to have to be extremely creative and resourceful in my efforts to visit Amy in Chicago as much as possible. With the war in Afghanistan continuing, March 2003 brought the invasion of Iraq. The United States military took Baghdad in relatively short order, and it wasn't long before I found myself traveling with Secretary Rumsfeld on his first trip to the region.

It was a big trip, and it seemed like every reporter who had ever stepped foot in the Pentagon wanted in. After we landed, Secretary Rumsfeld and his staff were put in armored Humvees for the trip into Baghdad. Meanwhile, all the traveling reporters were herded onto a big bus that would trail behind the secretary's caravan. Inexplicably to me, the one, singular, defining characteristic of the press bus they had for us was that it seemed to be made entirely of glass. I mean glass glass. Not any of that multilayered, high-tech, bulletproof stuff, either. Perfect for getting a good view riding into Baghdad, but perhaps not the safest vehicle for a war zone.

There we were, just a few days after U.S. troops took Baghdad, and it was as if someone in the DOD press shop came up with the brilliant idea that this might be the perfect opportunity for an American Journalists on Parade float that could be seen for miles around as if we were practicing for the Macy's Thanksgiving Day Parade. We were so visible—and vulnerable—from

a distance I was convinced we looked like we were in a giant goldfish bowl on wheels headed straight down the airport road for the Baghdad aquarium.

Before we departed, a young Army captain on the bus mumbled something about helmets and flak jackets being in the back for anyone who wanted them. I don't know if we didn't hear him clearly, if he didn't like the press, or if it was simply war-zone machismo, but not one reporter on the bus went for a helmet or a flak jacket.

Despite being in the middle of a war zone, the reporters on the bus were all in pretty high spirits, and everyone was busting each other out over one thing or another. Soon I could hear some crackling on the radio up near the front of the bus. It was very difficult to make out exactly what was being said, but I clearly heard the words "Humvee," "shots," and "SECDEF."

None of my colleagues on the bus seemed to notice or care what I was hearing on the radio. Finally, I spoke up and asked the driver if, indeed, I heard correctly that one of Secretary Rumsfeld's Humvees had been shot at.

"Yes," the driver answered nonchalantly. "The Secretary's Humvee took a few bullets."

Immediately, everyone—and I mean everyone—in that floating fishbowl, veteran and rookie alike, jumped out of their seats and dove toward the previously ignored pile of helmets and flak jackets in the rear of the bus.

By the time we arrived at Baghdad's Green Zone, all the reporters on that bus were more than ready to jump out of the goldfish tank and into the nearest restroom to compose themselves.

It was during this same trip that I started bonding with some of my fellow defense reporters who worked

for other networks. Despite the intense day-to-day competition that takes place among reporters covering the same beat, there always seems to be plenty of camaraderie to balance things, especially on overseas trips when you are stuck on planes or hanging in the same hotel lobbies for hours. Covering Defense Secretary Rumsfeld on this trip to Iraq was no exception.

Being fairly new to the Pentagon beat I found myself increasingly hanging around two long-time defense correspondents, NBC's Jim Miklaszewski and Jack McWethy of ABC. Jack was a fellow graduate of DePauw University, so he sort of took it upon himself to show me the ropes when I first arrived at the Pentagon. Both great guys and fantastic reporters, one of the things we all had in common was our love of golf.

During this particular trip to Iraq, we had a one-day stopover in Doha, Qatar. Being inveterate golfers and always looking for new courses to play during our downtime in Doha, Jack, Jim, and I decided to try to play a round at the course where they hold the Doha Masters, a huge event in that part of the world.

Knowing our very tight schedule covering the defense secretary, the folks at the course couldn't have been nicer. They got us fixed up with some clubs and a cart for a quick round of golf on this spectacular spring day. Everything was going great. Fantastic weather. Fun conversation. Some serious male bonding going on, and just a wonderful time hanging with these veteran reporters I had admired from afar for so many years.

Once on the eighth hole of the course, however, I received a phone call from my producer telling me that Secretary Rumsfeld had decided to hold an unscheduled news conference in his hotel in forty-five minutes. If

we dropped everything and hustled we would be able to make it in just enough time to get to the briefing.

The call ended and I said, "Guys, we gotta go."

Quite indignant, both Jim and Jack looked at me like I was absolutely crazy, insisting we finish our eighteen holes at this once-in-lifetime world-class golf course.

"Secretary Rumsfeld is having a press conference. We have to go," I insisted.

Jack and Jim were equally insistent that Rumsfeld would say nothing of news value and our time would be much better spent continuing our game. My companions might have been legends in the news business, but I was just this brand-new beat reporter still trying to find my way. I didn't exactly have any laurels to speak of, let alone anything to fall back on when I told my bosses I decided to play a round of golf instead of attending a news conference with the one man on the planet they happened to be paying me to cover.

"You guys can finish the round, but I have to go," I said, with some amount of authority.

Jack and Jim reluctantly decided to leave with me. We raced to get to the hotel in time for the news conference. Jack and Jim were both convinced Secretary Rumsfeld would make zero news that day, but I had my marching orders. The trip from the course to the hotel was filled with world-class moaning by these legendary reporters who were fully convinced the briefing would be a complete waste of time.

With just a minute to spare, we arrived at the hotel where the press briefing was being held. Secretary Rumsfeld came out and proceeded to take a sum total of three questions. And, of course, he made no news at all.

We dutifully pressed Rumsfeld on a couple of issues,

but he said absolutely nothing of news value, and the session ended as quickly as it began.

After the news conference was over, Jack and Jim quickly descended on me with some very condescending looks.

"We could have been on the fourteenth hole by now," Jim said.

I heard about that episode the entire rest of the trip, not to mention during a very long plane ride back home to the United States.

After being back in Washington for a few weeks, I continued to plot all kinds of new ways to impress Amy and convince her I was the guy for her. As we approached May and Amy's birthday on the seventh, it hit me. I had been invited by General Richard Myers to attend a dinner in Washington for the incoming NATO defense ministers and top military generals. Seven Central and Eastern European countries had been accepted into NATO, and the general was throwing a fancy dinner for them at Washington's Russia House. Only one of two reporters invited to attend the event, I was told I could bring a guest.

"Perfect!" I thought.

I could fly Amy into town, wow her with this impressive Washington dinner, and then whisk her out on the town for a big birthday celebration to finish the evening. In the meantime, I would be able to seed my contact list with names and numbers of the defense ministers and all the top brass from Estonia, Latvia, Lithuania, Slovenia, Slovakia, Bulgaria, and Romania. This was going to be great; how could this not impress Amy?

Having emptied the Silver Bullet of every last article of clothing remaining from the dirty laundry episode, I

picked Amy up at Reagan National and we drove directly to the dinner. Amy looked stunning!

Wearing a beautiful red dress and gold evening shoes that took her to new heights, Amy was about a quarter inch above me at five feet eleven. Despite the height difference, everything about this evening was going to be perfect. I escorted Amy into Russia House, where Chairman of the Joint Chiefs General Myers and his wife, Mary Jo, greeted us at the front door. I introduced Amy to them, and I could see she was duly impressed. I thought to myself, "Everything is going according to plan."

After greeting General and Mrs. Myers, Amy and I proceeded to a small table where a smartly uniformed woman officer gave us our seating assignments. The officer picked up two small envelopes and said, "Mr. Baier, you're at the chairman's table, table one. And Ms. Hills, you are with the defense minister of Estonia, at table number eight."

Amy looked horrified. I turned to the officer and said, "I'm sorry, there must be some kind of mistake. We should be together at the same table."

The officer calmly and kindly said, "No sir. All couples are split up. The chairman likes the interaction this way."

Not only could I see the apprehension on Amy's face, I saw my perfectly planned "seal the deal" dinner date going up in smoke. I had brought Amy to this fancy dinner with the incoming members of NATO thinking we would be sitting together. I hadn't briefed her on anything.

It was a little too late for me to come up with a briefing paper filled with bullet points of witty and hu-

morous things to drop in during a two-hour dinner conversation about Estonian defense capabilities. I was subjecting Amy to the defense minister and all the military brass from Estonia, a country that ninety-nine percent of the brilliant people in Washington wouldn't be able to find on a wall map even if they had Alex Trebek standing next to them holding a laser pointer. Images of my life passed before my eyes as I envisioned Amy having to sit through two hours of broken-English diatribes on the threat from Iran, strong-armed Russian energy policy, and specifics about Estonian troop movements in Afghanistan—all on her birthday, no less.

"Wow, did I really screw this up," I mumbled to myself.

After General Myers offered an opening toast to the new members of NATO, the dinner was underway. While I did my best to make smart and "fair and balanced" dinner conversation at the chairman's table, the entire time I was glancing over my shoulder to table number eight. Oddly, every time I sneaked a peak across the room toward Amy, I could see everyone at her table was laughing, giggling, even guffawing. Finally, I couldn't stand it anymore. I excused myself to use the restroom, strategically swinging by Amy's table on the way.

I introduced myself to the Estonian defense minister and the other brass at the table. In a very thick Estonian accent, the defense minister said, "Your girlfriend is beautiful and *very* entertaining. We are having wonderful time!"

I said thank you, then leaned in and whispered in Amy's ear, "Are you okay? What in the world are you all talking and laughing about?"

Amy whispered back, "They started out asking me what I thought about Russia joining NATO, and I said I hadn't formed my thoughts on that yet. Amy said every time they asked her a specific political or military question, she simply turned it around on them and steered the conversation to areas she was comfortable with: Broadway, fashion, travel, television shows. Anything other than Estonian politics, defense capabilities, or the million other topics I feared she would be pressed about during the entire dinner.

"They're very nice," Amy said, as if she were talking about some long-lost uncles she was having a beer with at Gibsons Steakhouse in Chicago. Amy Hills from Chicago was just fine—*Thank you very much!*—hobnobbing with all these VIPs and military brass from Estonia after I provided her with zero advance notice.

I already knew Amy was the one for me, exceeding all the categories on any checklist I had ever come up with. But there she was, owning the table at this high level, diplomatic affair deep in the trenches of Washington, D.C., and she seemed to be having the time of her life. There wasn't even a checklist category for how she handled herself that night.

As the dinner wrapped up, I leaned over and asked General Myers and his deputy, Marine General Peter Pace, for a favor. As we were getting ready to leave and Amy said good-byes to her new friends from Estonia, with all eyes in the room on them, General Myers and General Pace marched over to where Amy and I were standing. Suddenly, two of the top military leaders in the country started singing "Happy Birthday" to Amy. It was a perfect ending to a dinner that had all the mak-

ings of being a hall-of-fame, relationship-ending disaster date.

With Operation Dirty Laundry and the Estonian Disaster Date now growing smaller in the rearview mirror, it wasn't long before Amy and I started talking seriously about getting married. As in other areas of her life, Amy knew exactly what she wanted when it came to a ring. So, secretly, I started to hunt it down for her.

By late fall, I could sense Amy was waiting for me to pop the big question. We took a trip to the Bahamas for a getaway weekend and had a blast. At dinner the first night, Amy busted out a sexy black dress and was also carrying a camera. Throughout the meal, she was staring at me and smiling with these expectant, adoring eyes. I thought, "Uh-oh. She thinks this is it."

Finally, after some long walks, romantic sunsets, those puppy dog eyes, and always with the camera, I told Amy, "Honey, I'm sorry. This is not the engagement." From that moment forward, the mood of the weekend changed dramatically and that camera never made it to another meal.

About a month after the Bahamas trip, my mom and brother were again in Naples, along with the entire Hills clan: Amy's parents, Paul and Barbie Hills, her older brother, Tom, and his wife, Darby, her twin brother, Danny, and her little brother, John Paul, known as J.P. I decided I would take everyone out to dinner two nights before Thanksgiving.

During the day, Amy and I walked by a jewelry store on the way to play tennis with her family. I looked in

the window and said, "Babe, that sure is a pretty ring there. What is your ring size again? I really need to get that right."

Red with anger, Amy turned to me and hollered, "You don't know my ring size after all this time? It's five and three quarters!"

The tennis match that followed was intense. Amy definitely had a little something extra on her backhand whenever she sent a ball sailing my way.

That evening we all went to the Grill at the Ritz-Carlton for dinner. During the meal, I excused myself from the table to take some phone calls from work. After dinner, the family went to the bar, where a band was playing and a few dozen people were out on the dance floor. Everyone in our group ordered drinks, and I looked at my phone and turned to Amy and said, "Sorry, babe, I'll be right back. Another work call."

By this time, Amy had a face similar to the one she'd had on the tennis court earlier in the day. After I left, Amy turned to her mom and said, "Bret totally blew it! He could have asked me right here with all of our family. This stinks!" All of a sudden, in the middle of Amy's meltdown, and me now away from the table, the band stopped playing and the lead singer said, "We have a special guest who would like to say a few words. Let's welcome Mr. Bret Baier!"

From behind the curtain just off the dance floor, I popped out wearing a tuxedo and took the microphone. I could see Amy was in complete shock.

"I'd like to ask the love of my life, Amy Hills, to come up to the dance floor, please," I said.

A spotlight found Amy at her seat and followed her as

she made her way to the center of the dance floor where I was standing.

"Only a few hours after I met you, I knew I wanted to marry you, and over the past year I have grown to love you more every day. You are everything I have ever wanted. You're my best friend, my soul mate, my love."

Pulling out the ring, I got down on one knee in the middle of that dance floor, and with the spotlight still shining, I said: "Amy Hills, will you marry me?"

Amy had her hands on her face, and with tears streaming she replied, "Yes! Yes! Yes!"

On cue, the band started playing what Amy and I had already decided was our song, "When You Say Nothing at All," by Allison Krauss. Amy kissed me as we danced and said, "I told my Mom you blew it. I guess I was wrong."

The rest of the family joined us on the dance floor for several more songs, and that celebration pretty much continued all the way to our wedding day in Chicago in October 2004. Almost two years to the day from our blind date at the Rolling Stones concert, Amy and I were married. Although we couldn't book the Stones for our reception, the wedding was everything Amy had ever envisioned. She looked like a princess. Seeing her come down the aisle, I had to take several deep breaths so I could keep it all together.

It was a big day for me for many reasons. I had been estranged from my father for a very long time after my parents divorced. So, with the rest of the family gathered for the big occasion, Amy and I were happy my dad was there to help us celebrate as we began our new life together.

Because of our D.C.-Chicago-Afghanistan-Iraq long-

distance relationship, our eight-day honeymoon on the Island of Hawaii was the most days we had ever spent together consecutively. During long walks on the beach we tried to predict where the big problem areas might be in the Baier-Hills cohabitation department.

"You put your toothbrush where?"

"You need all that time to get ready?"

"What's a hamper?"

"Yes, that's my favorite football sweatshirt! It stays!"

Amy and I had purchased a condo in Georgetown preconstruction, and workers were still finishing up projects around the place until just a few hours before we moved in. With barely enough time to pull it off, I lit a few candles, placed some flowers on the counter, and met Amy at the elevator. At 4:47 p.m. on a windy October afternoon in Washington, I carried my completely adorable, gold-medal neat-freak dream girl from Chicago—*my wife*—across the threshold and into our first home at 3303 Water Street in Georgetown. By 4:48 p.m. I was happily enrolled in Amy's graduate-level continuing education course on the nuances and intricacies of "a thing for every place, and a place for every thing."

CHAPTER THREE

Complicated Heart

Winds of change were blowing across the National Mall and all through Washington in January 2007. After twelve years of Republican control, not only did Democrats win back the House of Representatives in the midterm elections, the nation got its first-ever woman Speaker of the House in Nancy Pelosi of California, a truly historic exchange of the gavel. While Speaker Pelosi and her colleagues were glorying in their expanded responsibilities and upgraded office space on Capitol Hill, the Baier condo in Georgetown was undergoing some pretty significant changes, too. The truly historic news around our house was the fact that Amy was pregnant with our first child, a boy.

Amy and I were over the moon with joy when we found out we were going to become parents. We both love children, and having a family was something we talked a lot about even before we got married. Obviously doing a little more than simply talking about it, Amy and I were equally nervous and excited when we learned the news. Any soon-to-be first-time parents

know the unique alchemy of extreme joy and severe trepidation that occurs as you anticipate the arrival of that first child.

It's one thing to be a young, fun couple with great jobs, friends, and family, living in an exciting town, going out to dinner every night, and all the rest. But during your late-night, alone times, all those things, as wonderful as they are, fade away when you realize not only are you bringing another human being into this world, you are personally responsible for that baby's survival and well-being. That stark dose of reality jolting you awake at three in the morning is the ultimate wake-up call for first-time parents. Having a baby—*our son*—was definitely the proverbial final frontier for us, but Amy and I had confidence we were up to the challenge and were really looking forward to becoming Mama and Papa Baier, no matter how daunting it sometimes seemed.

About the same time Amy and I were contemplating our big step into the world of parenting, more news landed on our doorstep. After I'd spent five years at the Pentagon, Fox News had officially named me the network's chief White House correspondent. Whether overtly or subliminally, I think I had been navigating toward the White House briefing room ever since my days at DePauw and Ken Bode's course on presidential politics. I had admired many White House reporters over the years, so being chosen by Fox to be part of that storied tradition was a great honor.

Although it was a logical professional leap for me to take across the Potomac from the Pentagon to the White House, that decision wasn't as easy as you might think. Over the past five years I had made something like twenty-three trips to Afghanistan and Iraq and had many

opportunities to meet some of the best, brightest, and bravest young people this nation has to offer. Talking to many of those soldiers who voluntarily and selflessly put themselves in harm's way for the rest of us had been a humbling and moving experience. It convinced me that the Greatest Generation should not be a designation reserved for heroes of the past. Even though I was definitely ready for a new career challenge to keep the professional juices flowing, I left the Pentagon beat with a fair amount of emotion. I was a changed person for having been there.

Now that I was fully embedded at the White House, and with Amy fully embedded with our first child, these were exciting days for us. Along with covering the final two years of the Bush presidency, apparently I was also going to have to read a few position papers on swaddling, diaper changing, and surviving on little or no sleep. Having been a journalist all of my adult life, I think I had number three pretty much nailed. But I was definitely going to need a few tutorials on points one and two on that list.

To be honest, I felt a little guilty having this huge new job at the White House at the same time my wife was going through her first pregnancy. But knowing how much I loved presidential politics, Amy supported me a hundred percent and was excited for me—*for us*. Commissioned with our marching orders for 2007, Amy and I both threw ourselves into our new responsibilities with as much energy as we could muster.

While I was still getting my legs under me at the White House, Amy was knocking it out of the park with her pregnancy. A little morning sickness here and there, but she seemed to take it all in stride, with few

complaints. Working out seven days a week, Amy was probably in the best shape of her life. She looked absolutely fantastic and definitely had the traditional glow of the expectant mother.

Not only was Amy doing great, but Paul Francis, named after Amy's dad, seemed to be coming along just fine, too. Every time Amy had a checkup or sonogram, the doctors told us everything looked perfect. No matter where you are on the planet or whatever your personal circumstances, all a new parent wants to know is if the baby is healthy—and ours was. We couldn't have been happier.

During one of Amy's early checkups a doctor thought he might have heard a slight heart echo, but we were relieved when he determined it was just a problem with the machine. We felt extremely blessed that all the indicators told us our son was perfectly healthy, right on schedule, and would be playing golf with me as soon as I could find him the right size clubs.

Early in the summer Amy bought the perfect child seat for the back of our car, and every time we drove around town and saw that empty seat we smiled, knowing it wouldn't be too many days before there would be a living, breathing little person sitting back there.

Activating the reliable and age-old through-the-belly communications network, every chance I got I would talk to Paul and tell him how exciting it was going to be to finally meet him. I strongly suggested it would be just fine with me if he wanted to hurry things up a little. Occasionally I even slipped in a few prodigy-nurturing tips on his yet-to-be-developed golf game. Excitement doesn't come close to describing my feelings as Amy's delivery date approached.

As we got closer to the date, like most couples, Amy and I worked out our plan for getting to the hospital when the time came. My car navigation system appropriately programmed for Sibley Hospital, and several dry runs under my belt, I was as prepared as any non-NASA mission controller could be. And just as if we were both working back in the Atlanta bureau, Amy and I had our go-bags packed and ready for the big day or night.

One night, thinking Amy might be going into labor, we made a hurried dash to Sibley, but it turned out to be a false alarm. Chalking it up to freshman jitters, we knew we were getting close, so we considered that trip a good dress rehearsal for the real thing, which we were convinced was just around the corner.

Then, one muggy Thursday evening after I got home from the White House, Amy and I went for one of our regular walks in our Georgetown neighborhood. One day earlier, Amy had experienced a few labor pains, but nothing like dress-rehearsal night. After we finished our walk and returned home, Amy started feeling like something newsworthy might be going on inside her. Right at the nine-month mark, this seemed like the real deal, so we decided to officially launch Operation Sibley.

After all my practice runs and having gone through the get-to-the-hospital scenario a thousand times in my head, I, of course, totally freaked. I started running around the condo like the proverbial headless chicken—pretty nervous, unprofessional stuff from someone who used to love driving directly into the path of hurricanes. Thankfully, Amy did stay calm and immediately started with her breathing exercises. This was a very good thing, because it helped me to remind her

to start with her breathing exercises. All packed up and ready to go to Sibley, we grabbed our bags and headed for the elevator.

Getting an early jump on the weekend, one of our condo neighbors had been having a late-night party. I remember hearing bass sounds thumping through the walls, not exactly the harmonious, serene music you might hope for at a time like this. On the other hand, maybe Paul heard the ruckus, thought it was his welcoming parade, and decided it might be a great time to make his grand entrance on planet Earth.

Still a little rattled by all the bass-thumping and just about everything else going on around me, I jumped on the elevator with my ready-to-pop, nine-months-pregnant wife, and here comes my party-throwing neighbor, Rob Jewell, who had no idea we were on our way to the hospital.

Rob, a great guy and super-successful dotcom entrepreneur, started to approach Amy with what appeared to me was going to be a huge, blubbering, party-style, frat-boy, body hug of an innocent neighborly greeting. Thinking that his impending bear hug just might pop Paul Francis out right there in that Otis elevator, I hollered, "Don't touch her. She's pregnant!"

We laughed about this later, but Rob immediately begged forgiveness, realizing he had invaded our not-so-calm departure for the hospital and Amy's delivery. Up to that point Rob's entrepreneurial claim to fame had been creating the highly successful website FreeCondoms.com. The irony of that elevator episode didn't hit me till later.

Despite my fears that our son might be born somewhere between the fourth and fifth floors of our condo

building, once we actually got to the Sibley delivery room Paul decided to play hard to get and take his good ole time about things. It was a very long night for Amy, and steering clear of the collective smirks and rolled eyes of an army of dues-paying mothers from coast to coast, I will refrain from uttering a single word about how long a night it was for me.

I have often thought if cosmic roles were reversed and men were the ones having babies, there would be national laws requiring us to be put into medically induced comas at about the third week of pregnancy, lasting through the delivery, past the diaper-changing years, and lasting to about the time our child was stepping onto the soccer field or baseball diamond for the first time.

Spirituality and sacredness of the moment temporarily aside, there's no way to sugarcoat it. Amy was having a very rough go of it there in the delivery room. Worrying. Eating ice chips. More worrying. Extreme pain. Praying. Waiting for the signal to push. More ice chips. False confidence from me. And then the entire cycle would repeat itself.

After several hours of this, Amy was finally told she could begin to push.

The numbers on Paul's heart monitor immediately started to drop, and I could see a level of concern on the doctors' faces. I was trying my best to project a cool, calm, everything-is-fine air of confidence for Amy to see, but that was a little difficult to do since the dial on my own worry meter had pegged into the red zone at about ice chip number two.

Suspecting Paul might be in a bad position for delivery or the umbilical cord might be kinked up, and with his heart rate still dropping, the doctors seriously consid-

ered performing a C-section. Suddenly, about a hundred twenty-seven separate things started happening at once, so there wasn't much time for me to whip out my press pass and start asking questions.

Everyone in the delivery room seemed to know exactly what their role in the choreography was, and eventually the doctors were successful in using a suction device to get Paul out without having to perform surgery. He was a bit purple and did cry a little, but it was nothing like the big booming stuff you see in the movies.

The doctors seemed somewhat concerned, but suddenly Paul's color improved and everyone in the room started breaking into big smiles.

Relief all around. Paul was now looking great and had a good steady heartbeat. The nurses placed Paul in Amy's arms and she started to cry. Then I started to cry. And now Paul started to cry, too. I remember thinking that delivery room cacophony sounded as sweet as any Brahms concerto ever performed.

The flood of emotions I felt at that moment was overwhelming. My son was finally here in this room, with us, right now, and there was nothing but love going on. Love for my son. Love for my wife. Love for our families and friends. Love for God. Love for anyone who helped us get to this sacred place, including Mick Jagger, Keith Richards, and all the Rolling Stones.

Amy and I had shared the most intimate experience this life has to offer, and there we were with our son, a life created because of Amy's love for me and mine for her. And now we, all three Baiers, were together at last. Simply spectacular.

The doctors in the room didn't seem particularly concerned about anything, but they decided to give Paul

a few tests. The nurses cleaned him up a bit and took him away for a few minutes. Before long our pediatrician came in and told us the only thing you ever want to hear—he said Paul was fine.

No problems. Ten fingers. Ten toes. Breathing well. Heart sounds good. Paul was perfect, head to toe. The range of emotions during the past ten to twelve hours had been extraordinary. But hearing that report from our pediatrician sent our souls to the top of Mount Everest. Our spirits could not have soared any higher.

Starting with Paul's birth at 12:34 p.m. on a Friday, June 29, 2007, the next twenty-four hours at Sibley were a wonderful, blissful blur of activity. Amy was perfectly fine to be alone in the room nesting with Paul, but being the newsman in the family I felt compelled to get this huge story out there.

So just a few hours after Paul's live shot audition in the Sibley delivery room, I sent my first news flash to family, friends, and Fox News colleagues:

June 29, 2007, 4:32 PM, Friday
Subject: It's the THREE Baiers NOW!!

Papa Baier, Mama Baier—and NOW…

Paul Francis Baier HAS ARRIVED! And he's just right.

He was born here in Washington at 12:34 PM at Sibley Hospital. He's 6 lbs., 12 oz., and 19 1/2 inches long.

Mama and Baby Baier are doing great…and Papa Baier is amazed at the whole process!

Thanks for all of your kind words and wishes.

Attached find a pic of Paul on his first day on earth.

Paul was staying with Amy and me right there in the room, and it was awesome. I felt like I was walking on air the entire time. Over the course of my career in journalism I had traveled on hundreds of trips to some really exotic locales all around the world, even some recent ones on Air Force One with the president of the United States. But I never, ever had more excitement flowing through me than I did that day as I anticipated spending the night with my wife and son in the cramped confines of our little nest of a room in the Sibley maternity ward.

Amy's mother and father, Barbie and Paul Hills, and her younger brother, J.P., flew in from Chicago to share in our joy and excitement. Everyone in the family wanted in on this huge story, and it was a wonderful time of taking photographs, holding Paul, and sharing our joy. Being with family and having my son right there in the room with us, I was truly counting my blessings.

The pure joy I had in my heart from meeting my son for the first time reminded me of an incident just a few years before during a trip I took to Afghanistan. At a Forward Operating Base with some soldiers just back from the fight along the Afghan-Pakistan border, I was sharing a computer room with a young soldier I had been with in the field for several days.

These were the earliest days of Skype and of being able to visually communicate real-time over the computer. While I was in the middle of writing up a news story for Fox, I couldn't help but see and hear the soldier

next to me being introduced to his newborn son for the first time right there on the computer. It was such a joyous and momentous event for him, he began to weep. Caught up in the moment I also began to tear up.

Thinking about that soldier, I realized that being able to be with my son physically during his first hours on earth and being surrounded by loving family members was a blessing not everyone enjoys. I had never been more grateful about anything in my entire life.

Also, on that first day at Sibley with Paul and Amy, I had a few opportunities to show off everything I had learned from all those position papers on swaddling and diaper changing. The swaddling went perfectly fine—it was even fun. But that first diaper change was—how to put this delicately—*disgusting*! There is no book, training session, or position paper that can prepare you for something like that. There were colors in that diaper I never imagined existed anywhere in the known universe.

Like any reporter faced with a totally unique story situation for the first time, I quickly started flipping mental pages to see if I could come across something—*anything*—from my experiences that might help me come to terms with what I was witnessing. Cleaning up an oil spill on any beach in the world would surely be better duty than this. The only reference point I could possibly use to gauge the primordial concoction before me was from one of those bloodcurdling scenes I remembered from the first time I saw the movie *Alien*.

Early Saturday morning, after the three Baiers' wonderful overnight Sibley campout, and having survived the premier performance of *The Diaper from Outer Space*, Paul apparently had some unfinished business down the hall when a nurse came to take him to be circumcised. I

went along for moral support but, looking down at Paul, and with all the courage I could muster, I whispered, "Sorry, pal." I have sometimes wondered if Paul's one-day's-worth of life experience ever suggested to him that this might be payback for that first diaper.

After the circumcision and when Paul was back in the room with us, Amy's folks returned, and it was picture-taking time all over again. Amy's dad, Paul Francis Hills, perhaps exercising the unwritten rights associated with having a grandson named after him, started calling the baby Paulie. We laughed about that, thinking *Goodfellas* and *The Sopranos* might have already cornered the Paulie market. But before long we were all calling our little guy Paulie. The naming rights came with a cost for Amy's dad, who immediately became either Big Paul or Franpa.

Paul—Paulie—was doing great, and so was Amy, who was seriously talking like she was ready to get out of there and reestablish this party back at the Georgetown condo. We had a spectacular room all spiffed up for Paulie, and since the nine-month lease on his old place had run out we couldn't wait to show him his new digs.

With mother and son doing so well, and being the attentive son-in-law I am, I offered to take Amy's folks to lunch and bring her something back from her favorite salad haunt, Sweet Green. While we were out I also wanted to show Amy's folks a house in the area we were looking at. So we left for a few hours, hoping Amy might be able to catch a nap while we were gone.

While we were away, things back at Sibley were fine, with one exception. The nurse assigned to Amy and Paulie had a seizure while on duty in the hospital. Everything turned out fine with her, but assignments

had to be shifted around, and Paulie and Amy now had a new nurse looking after them. Entering the room to check on mother and baby for the first time, nurse Beth Kennedy took one look at Paul and said she thought his color seemed off.

Amy and I were brand-new parents who had just met Paulie for the first time less than twenty-four hours before. We had no idea what his normal color was supposed to be. We did notice Paulie didn't seem too interested in Amy's milk that morning, but we were told that was fairly normal after a circumcision.

Beth suggested to Amy that Paulie's pale color might be the result of some kind of bacterial infection. She thought he should have a few tests just to be safe. So she took him to the hospital's Neonatal Intensive Care Unit (NICU) so he could be checked out. Amy called to fill me in on the possible bacterial infection. After dropping her folks off at their hotel, I returned to Sibley.

I was back in the room with Amy for a short while when Beth came in to let us know the bacterial infection tests had all come back negative. This was a huge relief. Amy had been told that newborns with any kind of bacterial infection often stay in the hospital for as many as ten additional days. After all the excitement of Paulie's birth and the wonderful overnight we had with him there in the room, Amy couldn't fathom the idea of leaving the hospital without her son, let alone not taking him home for another ten days.

While Amy and I were thrilled with the news that Paulie didn't have an infection, Nurse Kennedy wasn't. Still concerned about his color, Beth told us she wanted to run some more tests and page a doctor to come in and take a look just to be safe.

Dr. Gerard Martin is the father of five children, all of whom played competitive soccer on one level or another. Trying to figure out which field he needed to be at on any given Saturday could sometimes be a challenge, and even more difficult on weekends when he was on call. This happened to be one of those weekends.

Even though Dr. Martin was a department head at Children's National Medical Center in Washington, he still had to do regular doctoring from time to time. On Saturday, June 30, 2007, he was doing just that. Dressed casually for some morning soccer games, Dr. Martin was already on his way to Georgetown Hospital in response to a page he received about a baby there who seemed to be having some issues.

As he drove from Chevy Chase toward Georgetown, Dr. Martin received a completely separate page from the Neonatal Intensive Care Unit at Sibley Hospital about a one-day-old they also had some concerns about—our Paulie. Sitting at a traffic light, Dr. Martin called the Sibley NICU back and was told they thought they heard a heart murmur and that Paulie was breathing faster than normal. They also expressed concern because they couldn't get a good pulse reading in his legs, possibly indicating some sort of blockage.

Based on what he was hearing, Dr. Martin made an instant decision, banked a right turn, and headed directly to Sibley. His gut already told him the Georgetown case was not as serious, but he had zero doubts about the situation at Sibley.

Dr. Martin was driving right past Sibley at the time he received the page, so he arrived there just a minute

or two later. Once at the NICU, he went right to work trying to find out what might be going on with his newest patient. Feeling Paulie's chest wall with his fingers, Dr. Martin noticed the heartbeat was much stronger than it should be—working way too hard for pumping blood through his little body. He continued listening and touching the baby's chest. Even as he prepared his young patient for an echocardiogram to get a more detailed look, Dr. Martin's instincts and thirty-plus years in cardiology already told him what was going on—and it wasn't good.

After hearing Paulie didn't have a bacterial infection, Amy and I were eager to get him back in the room with us so we could continue with that warm and wonderful Three Baiers bonding process. Amy was enjoying the salad I brought her from Sweet Green, and the mood in the room was upbeat as I filled her in on what her folks had to say about the house I took them to see.

Amy was a little miffed at me for being gone so long and not around to help her deal with the nurse reassignment issue and the bacterial infection scare. I reminded my dear wife I was out with *her* parents and not exactly quaffing beer with the boys at the nineteenth hole after playing a round of golf.

Amy, of course, knew that. But I realized then how worried she had been about the possibility of not being able to take Paulie home for ten more days. She was so looking forward to that day—*tomorrow*—when we would finally be able to put Paulie into the empty car

seat that we had been goofily grinning at for the past two months.

Amy is an incredibly strong person, both in mind and spirit. I could see in her eyes there was nothing that was going to keep her from taking her son home tomorrow. Upon hearing an infection might keep Paulie in the hospital one extra minute, I would not have been surprised if she didn't simply will—or pray—that bad boy of a possibility completely off Paulie's medical chart.

Now that she'd been told there was no infection, we sat there confident that whatever these extra precautionary tests were, Beth Kennedy would soon be coming in to tell us what we already knew: Paulie was perfectly healthy.

Over the years, I had done several stories about the mountain of medical litigation cases hospitals face every year. If they needed to run a few extra tests on Paulie so they could dot all their i's and cross all their t's to keep their lawyers happy, that was perfectly fine with me. There was nothing to worry about. We spent the entire night with Paulie right there in the room with us and there were no problems of any kind. Still, we were a little anxious about the situation. We chalked it up to having a new nurse who was probably just being abundantly cautious.

With the lights in the room down low so Amy could nap, I slipped out to the nurses' station to ask why it was taking so long for Paulie to get back. The nurses assured me it wouldn't be much longer, so I returned to the room to be with Amy.

Before long we heard a knock on the door and a doctor came in. He was someone we'd never laid eyes on before. Wearing civilian clothes, he apologized for

not looking the part, explaining his children were soccer players and he had been to a couple of games earlier in the day. With that, Dr. Gerard Martin introduced himself as the cardiologist who received the call from Sibley to come take a look at Paulie. Amy was lying down and I was sitting on the edge of the bed as Dr. Martin entered the room and flipped on the overhead lights.

"I need to talk to you about your son," he said.

The instant those harsh, clinical overhead lights came on I immediately got a sickening feeling of dread in the pit of my stomach, like playtime was over and I was now in the principal's office. Only this time it wasn't about me. This wasn't even about my wife, who was still recovering from giving birth one day before. This was about our one-day-old son.

My mind was racing two hundred miles per hour and in fifty different directions at once. Now operating on a seven-second delay, I realized Dr. Martin had introduced himself to us as a cardiologist. Why would a cardiologist be talking to us about a bacterial infection or the results of some precautionary tests?

My heart dropped as I started to put two and two together. I knew instantly and instinctively this was going to be exponentially worse than simply having to keep Paulie in the hospital for an extra ten days because of an infection. I quickly rewound the tape in my mind, now hoping that Paulie actually *did* have an infection.

Ten extra days? No problem! Keep him for twenty if you need to. We can deal with that. Piece of cake. Keep him as long as you need him. Let's just get our boy home healthy. An infection is nothing. Happens all the time. Please God, let Paul have this bacterial infection.

It's amazing the number of thoughts your mind can process and the speed at which it can process them in that frozen split second of a moment when you realize the comfortable reality you have known your entire life is over and you are now entering a place of uncertainty and fear from which you may never return.

I looked at Amy and she had sheer terror in her eyes. I moved closer and held her hand as Dr. Martin continued to speak. In a very calm but serious voice he said, "Your baby has heart disease. Heart disease can be simple or it can be complex. Your son has a complex heart disease. He has a *very* complicated heart."

That sentence hung there in the room as Amy and I sat silently on the bed in complete shock. Dr. Martin pulled out a piece of paper and started to draw a picture and talk at the same time. "Paulie's heart is built wrong," he said.

"The normal heart pumps this way, but Paulie's heart is pumping this way," indicating the exact opposite direction than the correct heart in his diagram.

"This is going to be a significant issue to deal with for a very long time," Dr. Martin said. "We do have ways to deal with it, but it is going to take some time to explain it all to you."

And then Dr. Martin uttered the words that have played in my mind on a continual loop every day since: "If your son doesn't have surgery within the next two weeks, he's not going to make it."

Immediately my mouth went completely dry. I didn't know where my next breath would come from. Time stopped. Unlike any moment I have experienced in my life, it resembled one of those slow-motion scenes in a

movie when you know the bomb is about to explode. Thoughts of complete doom filled my mind.

I remember squeezing Amy's hand, but my whole body was weightless. For a minute everything got completely fuzzy. I simply could not believe what I was hearing. Both of us were in a state of shock and disbelief. Neither Amy nor I said a word. My mind immediately started to flood with a torrent of discordant thoughts and questions for this doctor we had met for the first time all of two minutes ago.

"Who do you think you are coming in here on your high horse and telling us such horrible news? How could you possibly know this about our son? Maybe you have Paulie mixed up with someone else. Our son is completely healthy. Everybody knows that. They told us that all through Amy's pregnancy. Our pediatrician told us Paulie was perfect there in the delivery room. That was just yesterday, for God's sake—don't you know anything? You are clueless. You don't know what you're talking about. My God, Paul stayed right here in this room with us last night, didn't they tell you that? We need another doctor here. My son will be coming through that door any second now. How dare you come in here and bring us this horrible news? You should be ashamed of yourself for scaring us like that. And turn those lights back off!"

I, of course, did not say any of those things out loud, but Dr. Martin could see our confusion and dismay. Holding each other on that hospital bed, Amy and I both started to cry at the same time. These were not the Mount Everest tears of joy we'd shared the day before in the delivery room. These were the tears of totally distraught, scared-to-death parents who at that moment

were convinced their baby boy was going to die. We felt totally hopeless and lost.

Just a few hours before, right here in this room, we had taken several joyous pictures of the family with everyone holding Paulie, sharing the euphoric excitement, joy, and promise that goes with any new birth. Everyone was joking around about how Paulie was going to be a great golfer like his dad. It was a wonderful time. The kind of moment that, as you are experiencing it, you just know you are going to remember forever.

And now this.

A nuclear bomb of emotion had just detonated in that very same room, and everything that took place prior to that moment was instantly vaporized: the memories, the laughs, the picture taking, everything. All those things were now obliterated in a mushroom cloud of despair. Now, none of that stuff meant anything. Paul had been with us less than thirty hours, and now his life was hanging in the balance. How could this possibly be happening?

In the midst of all the sadness, grief, and torment of that moment—*the worst moment of my life*—it was almost like I started to have some kind of out-of-body experience. Through the tears and the numbness, I began to hear words coming out of my mouth. Probably out of sheer desperation and helpless panic knowing I had no control over anything at that moment, my journalism training started to kick in, and I began with what must have been a million questions for Dr. Martin: "How can you have all this information after being with Paulie less than thirty minutes? Does Paulie need to have surgery today? Can he get this fixed right here at Sibley? What happens if they operate and can't fix the problem?

Where should we go for the surgery? Who's the best in the country, the world, for doing the kind of surgery he needs? When can we fix this?"

Finally, just as I would do if I heard a newsmaker make an outlandish claim that demanded to be followed up, I reframed Dr. Martin's bombshell sentence to make sure I heard him correctly: "So you're saying if Paulie doesn't have surgery, he is going to die?"

I scared myself even more when I heard those stark words come out of my mouth. Dr. Martin replied, "Yes. Paulie has at least four, maybe five, separate congenital heart defects. He has a very, very complex heart." He went on to tell us Paulie would need at least one open-heart surgery—possibly more.

While I was reloading with a second barrage of technical and medical questions, Amy's motherly instincts kicked in and all she wanted to know was where Paulie was and if he was okay. Could she see him? Could she hold him?

Dr. Martin told us Paulie was in the NICU and was fine for the time being. He said he had given Paulie medication to stabilize him and keep his blood vessels open and flowing. Dr. Martin also explained that when a baby has heart disease like Paulie's, there is also an increased likelihood other abnormalities could exist in other internal organs. He told us the medication he gave Paulie would buy them some time so they could get a better, fuller read on the totality of what he might be facing.

I asked Dr. Martin what the next step was, and he told us he had already notified the cardiology department at Children's National Medical Center in D.C. He wanted Paulie transferred to Children's immedi-

ately so a team of specialists could assess the situation and start coming up with options for going forward. In fact, Paulie's case was so serious that even before Dr. Martin came into the room to talk to us he'd already called for a special cardiac transport team to come to Sibley to take him to Children's Cardiac Intensive Care Unit (CICU).

Dr. Martin explained that while Amy stayed at Sibley to continue recovering, I would need to follow the ambulance to Children's and take care of all the admissions paperwork there. Because of Paulie's complex and multiple issues, Dr. Martin told us they would need overnight to sort things out, and we would meet again in the morning over at Children's after he had more information.

Before he left the room, Dr. Martin told me that when the cardiac team arrived I would need to sign some papers so they could legally transport Paulie to Children's. In the meantime, we called Amy's folks at their hotel. Along with Amy's brother, they immediately hopped in a cab so they could return to Sibley to be with us. I also called my mother in Florida, who told me she was on her way.

After Dr. Martin left and we had made our phone calls, Amy and I were alone in the room. We looked at each other with tear-filled eyes and then held on to each other for dear life. Our world was spinning out of control, and neither one of us knew how to make it stop. We were both in a state of shock, disbelief, confusion, and fear over the possibility of losing our dear and precious son.

Raised as Catholics, Amy and I were both people of faith. But to be honest, at that very moment I had seri-

ous doubts God was on the job. As with my unspoken rant against Dr. Martin when he first told us of Paulie's condition, I did not have the guts to say out loud what my heart was now screaming: "Why us, Lord? Why did this have to happen to us? Things were going so great for us. Why did you do this to us?"

From the moment I laid eyes on Amy five years before, all the way through Paulie's birth, everything had been absolutely perfect for us. We fell in love. We got married. We bought a great condo on the water's edge in Georgetown. I had gone from being an unknown reporter, to Pentagon correspondent, to chief White House correspondent for Fox News.

I was traveling all over the world on Air Force One with the president of the United States. I loved working at Fox and the network was doing great. Amy and I were a very happy couple. We had everything going for us—had all we needed. Our hopes, dreams, and future prospects were unlimited. Everyone said so.

But now, none of that meant a thing.

There was only one reality now; our son was extremely sick, and there was a good chance he was going to die. Starting tomorrow morning we were going to have to begin making critical life-and-death decisions for *our son*. That was the only thing that mattered in our lives right now. In that moment, and in that hospital room, it became clear that this wasn't about me anymore. Not about career, money, or our cool place on the river.

My one-day-old son was getting ready to be strapped into the back of an ambulance without his mother or father to hold his hand for a trip across town to a strange place. That singular image of Paulie alone in

the back of an ambulance racing through the streets of D.C. to a hospital I never heard of immediately crashed the pity party I had been holding for myself. Paulie needed a clear-thinking father right now, and if I was going to be of any help at all to him I better man up—and quick.

All my life I had heard the saying "All things happen for a reason, even if you sometimes don't know why." I always thought that was one of those convenient phrases you plopped down on troubled souls from the comfort of the first-class cabin 35,000 feet up when you had minimal interest or nothing else to offer. Now, the sobering truth of that phrase landed front and center before Amy and me and bounced right up into our laps. As we sat there in that hospital room sobbing hopelessly in each other's arms, Amy and I both got a glimpse of the new realities and responsibilities about to overtake our lives.

Whether because of years of churchgoing or simply sheer desperation of two lost souls not knowing what else to do, right there in that hospital room, all by ourselves, with no pretense and no one watching, Amy and I held hands and began to pray.

We begged God to spare our son's life. We also asked him to give us strength and wisdom to be the kind of parents our son needed right now. Complicated heart or not, Paulie was God's special gift to us. Now it was our time to rise to the occasion and become the parents he needed and deserved to help him through the dark days ahead.

CHAPTER FOUR

Through the Storm

Still stunned by the chain of events that had overtaken us over the past sixty minutes, after we prayed together Amy threw on a robe and we headed out the door and down the hall toward Sibley's Neonatal Intensive Care Unit. While my brain was still trying to process all the medical information about Paulie's heart condition and details about transferring him to Children's National Medical Center, Amy had one goal: to get to her son. She needed to see him. Speak to him. Touch him. Hold him.

With my voracious appetite for news and information of all kinds, Amy knew me well enough to let me take the lead in asking the doctors and nurses most of the questions about Paulie's medical condition and the logistics for getting him to Children's. But I knew Amy well enough to know that even though Sibley's NICU was probably not the best place for a family reunion, there wasn't anything or anyone who was going to keep her from getting to her son at that moment, no matter where in the hospital he happened to be.

I am not sure she even knew where she was headed, but driven by her natural instincts and newly acquired motherly intuition, it was almost as if Amy had an internal GPS device guiding her exactly where she needed to go. Even though she was still in a fair amount of physical pain from giving birth the day before, it took everything I had to keep up with her, drafting in Amy's wake like I was trying to stay with Jimmie Johnson on the third turn at Talladega.

Having seen this headstrong mother-to-baby hospital quickstep before, the Sibley nurses and aides seemed to know instinctively what was going on and made a path for us as we walked by. Clogged corridors magically cleared as if we were the leads in a choreographed long hallway tracking shot in a high-budget Hollywood feature film. Unfortunately, the lighthearted romantic comedy we thought we were in just a few minutes ago had now jumped into the world of horror, with a very scary script and an uncertain ending.

The last time we were physically together in the room with Paulie our reality was that he was a perfectly healthy baby boy whose color seemed to be a little off and who wasn't eating much. "No big deal," I thought. Going through the process of childbirth, for mother and baby, is traumatic whether there are medical issues or not. To my untrained eye, it had seemed perfectly understandable that it might take a day or two for Paulie to get his full Baier mojo on. "Let's just get him home, and I am sure things will sort themselves out," I thought. One nurse even suggested that scenario earlier in the morning when we mentioned Paulie didn't seem too hungry.

Unfortunately, that armchair diagnosis turned out to be a little off the mark.

Now, when we looked down on Paulie for the first time after our bombshell meeting with Dr. Martin, it would be very tough envisioning the Masters golf champion or Super Bowl quarterback we'd joked about just a few hours before. Instead, we would be gazing down on an extremely fragile intensive care patient with multiple life-threatening heart defects—our precious six pound fourteen ounce one-day-old baby boy, Paul Francis Baier.

It was extremely difficult to comprehend the turn of events, and my head was swimming with fear and anxiety as Amy and I entered the wing leading to Sibley's NICU. All our excitement about taking Paulie home for the first time, getting him set up in his new room, midnight feedings, family vacations, first day in school, holidays, picnics, soccer games, golfing with his dad, and just about everything else we dreamed about over the past nine months would have to be put on hold for a while. And if we heard Dr. Martin correctly and didn't catch a serious break or two along the way, those hopes and dreams could very well slip away forever.

It was so early and there were still so many unknowns, even Dr. Martin couldn't say precisely what direction things might go, especially given the highly complex nature and abnormalities of Paulie's heart. Even if we caught that huge break and Paulie made it through a difficult open-heart surgery, would he ever be healthy enough to live the active life of a normal little boy? Would he have to spend his entire childhood on the sidelines? No one had answers for any of those questions.

Don't get me wrong. If that was the cosmic deal being

offered—Paulie survives but is very limited in what he can do—I would sign that contract one thousand out of a thousand times. I wouldn't have been thrilled about it, but I would have taken that deal in a proverbial New York minute.

The pure joy and excitement of those first twenty-four hours in the room with Paulie were enough to convince me this little guy was going to—actually already had—changed my life forever. Touching his flourlike skin. Running my index finger through his tiny fingers and toes. Feeling him breathe in and out as I held him against my chest. Watching his eyes open and try to focus on me as I uttered the most ridiculous things using the most ridiculous voices. But most of all, seeing Amy light up as if God himself had pumped pure sunshine into her soul whenever someone in the family would pass Paulie back to her to hold. It was pure bliss. And selfishly, I admit, I craved more golden moments just like that with the two people I loved more than anyone on this earth—Amy and Paulie.

Of all the scenarios swirling around my head as we walked, the scariest, of course, was the very real possibility Paulie might not even make it home from the hospital. Dr. Martin didn't sugarcoat any of that for us. Although he was very compassionate and caring in the way he spoke to us, he didn't dance around the real possibility that Paulie simply might not make it.

Forget soccer practice, trips to the golf course, or wrestling on the couch on a lazy Sunday afternoon. We could very well be dealing with a situation where Paulie continued to grow weaker and weaker by the hour and did not even make it to open-heart surgery, let alone survive it. I didn't dare share my dark introspections with

Amy, but by the look in her eyes I suspected she might have been having similar thoughts.

Thinking back on our conversation with Dr. Martin, I wondered—hoped, actually—that he might have laid out the obligatory worst-case scenario about congenital heart defects just so the hospital would be covered if things didn't go our way. Given the litigious world in which we live, doctors have to be extremely careful how they phrase things, especially when talking to desperate parents looking for the slightest glimmer of hope that their child will be one of the survivors.

My gut told me Dr. Martin was being completely straight with us, but every person and patient is unique. No one could say with certainty how an individual case will turn out. Medical professionals can quote facts and statistics about survivability rates until the cows come home. But with Paulie's situation there were just too many variables to consider, especially this early in the game.

It's not that I didn't trust what Dr. Martin was telling us, but after Amy's "flawless" pregnancy and having been told without equivocation in the delivery room that Paulie was perfect, I have to admit the needle on my Who–Can–I–Trust meter was bouncing all over the place. After all, if a sonogram missed Paulie's heart problems at Amy's thirty-seven-week checkup, who's to say Sibley's machines weren't out of whack, too? Maybe there was a glitch in all the machines and Paulie was perfectly healthy. This might turn out to be one of those happy-ending stories we bore all the relatives with at family gatherings for the next fifty years.

I knew if I worked this story long enough I could figure it all out and save the day for my son. What a great

news story: Flawed Medical Tests—Thousands of Sick Children Really Healthy. I might even get Fox to roll a satellite truck up North Capitol Street to Children's so I could do some live shots. I wondered if O'Reilly would be interested in my huge exposé. I was sure I could get Greta Van Susteren on it.

Now in a grade A government issue Psychology 101 classic state of denial, my mind was beginning to wander all over the crazy parts of the playing field.

I was desperately searching for any explanation other than the one staring me right in the face. My son was desperately ill, and there wasn't a thing I could do about it.

Unfortunately, Dr. Martin's reputation and medical pedigree were unquestioned, so I knew the Flawed Medical Tests story and any number of other ones my mind had conjured up were completely irrational. Still, with all the conflicting information of the past twenty-four hours, I really wasn't sure whom I should believe.

I knew these unspoken inner thoughts were negative and could be extremely counterproductive if I didn't hold them in check. I sure didn't want Amy to pick up on any of them. She was having a rough enough time being separated from Paulie, and I didn't want to do or say anything that would add to her stress level.

So I sucked it up and kept those thoughts to myself, hoping that even though Paulie's condition went undiagnosed for nine months, everyone now on the job was performing at the highest level and doing exactly what they were supposed to be doing.

Although I was truly thankful they discovered Paulie's heart condition while we were still there in the hospital, I could not stop thinking about what might have hap-

pened if Nurse Beth Kennedy hadn't come into our room exactly when she did. As we continued racing to Paulie, my mind was also racing and flashing some pretty horrible images. What if we had gone through normal discharge procedures, taken Paulie home, then spent a day or two—or even a week—trying to diagnose what might be going on with him?

I mean, after all, babies have eating issues all the time. And who's really to say what a newborn's perfect color should be? What if we had gotten Paulie home and a few days later woke up in the middle of the night to find him blue in the crib and struggling to breathe? No matter how we might have diagnosed why Paul wasn't eating or why his color was off, in a million years I would never have suspected something as serious as congenital heart disease. It's just not something you think about.

Deciding that the "what is" scenario was scary enough without conjuring up the "what if's," I tried my best to put the dark and negative thoughts out of my mind. But I simply could not get my brain around the idea that something as serious as heart disease wouldn't be picked up long before now. Safe to say I wasn't feeling any Tony Robbins optimism about the medical establishment at that particular moment, and I was definitely going to need a little time to sort things out and let my anger subside.

My entire life I have always been a positive, glass-half-full kind of guy. I have always been sold on the idea that sending out positive, uplifting vibes is not only a good way to live your life, it also brings good vibes back your way.

I totally bought into the universal principles of the

Secret, the Power of Positive Thinking, Paying It Forward, and the Golden Rule. When I was working at Hilton Head, I think I must have listened to every Tony Robbins tape ever recorded while I jogged on the beach one summer. But as I continued to think about Paulie and the enormous crisis he was facing, negative thoughts flooded my mind no matter how positive I tried to be. And I couldn't stop any of them.

I don't know if it's because I am a working journalist or simply just the way guys are wired to process information, but when I am hit with multiple challenges at the same time, I can normally place each of them into separate compartments in my mind: react to the ones that need immediate attention, hold back on the ones I have time to reflect on, prioritize, categorize, sequence. And always—*always*—keep the counterproductive drama to a minimum.

But the situation with Paulie was like nothing I had ever experienced. Suddenly, there were no boundaries. No compartments. No place to put anything. Everything I was sensing, feeling, and thinking was competing for my attention at exactly the same time and with equal intensity. I was having an extremely difficult time trying to distinguish between number one on the priority list and number 234.

Everything Dr. Martin told us back in the room was numbing and overwhelming. As Amy and I walked to the NICU we simply had no idea what we should expect for Paulie, or even what we could realistically hope for. I had no idea if I dared think beyond two or three weeks, let alone two or three years down the road.

Would a few years with Paulie be too much to ask?

At first it was simply one of a dozen questions racing

across the screen of my mind as we continued to make our way to our baby. But soon it slowed to a crawl and seemed to hang there all by itself. I knew Dr. Martin was in no position to offer any guarantees on that particular question or any of the other ones I had about Paulie's future.

"Dear Lord, would it be too much to ask to have a few years with Paulie? Please let me see my boy grow up. I have so much to tell him—so much to teach him!"

The fact that the question spontaneously morphed itself into a prayer surprised me. Raised a Catholic and having served as an altar boy back at All Saints Catholic Church in Atlanta, I was well aware of the rituals, doctrine, and tradition of the Church. But no matter how many times I served Mass or how many years I attended Catholic schools, it wasn't like I was someone who walked around quoting Bible verses or shooting up prayers to God every time I encountered a challenge in my life.

Given the seriousness of Paulie's situation and the intense personal nature of what we were experiencing, deep within me it seemed as if an inner voice was reminding me that prayer is simply talking to God whenever and wherever you happen to be during your moment of need. There were no stained glass windows or cushioned kneelers anywhere to be found in that Sibley hallway. Yet because of the urgency of our schedule and the dire situation in which we found ourselves, I figured if God was genuinely in the business of listening to heartfelt prayers from desperate souls—and I surely was one—then that busy corridor was as good a place as any to try to get something going in the miracle department for my son. I wasn't sure I if could hit

God up for the full monty and ask him to wipe the slate clean and zap Paulie with a brand-new, problem-free heart. But I thought two or three years was not an unreasonable place to start.

When we finally arrived at the NICU, I was a little surprised to see that the cardiac transport team from Children's was already there and prepping Paulie for his transfer. Their presence reinforced in my mind how serious Paulie's case must be. Moving with professional speed and precision, from across the room the transport team paramedics appeared to be like those white-robed technicians you see in grainy old NASA videos showing last-minute preparations before launching Apollo astronauts into space. No matter how professional or experienced the members of that team were, being forced to stand off to the side and watch several people we didn't know fidgeting around our son as though he was the center of the universe was surreal.

The paramedics gave the impression they had performed this kind of transfer a thousand times before. All good, but unfortunately when you are a parent in an intensive care unit and it is your son or daughter being wired up, you are not necessarily thinking about the thousand times the professionals have performed the procedure without a mistake. Given your totally stressed-out frame of mind, you are more than likely thinking this will be the one time in a thousand they really screw things up. Such is the anxiety level for any parent or loved one who has ever had to put in time around an intensive care unit or hospital waiting room, pediatric or otherwise.

I felt so bad for Amy. The mother of a newborn is emotionally and physiologically wired to be snuggling

with her baby—especially a one-day-old—with minimal distractions from the outside world. Now it seemed that the entire outside world was hovering around Paulie, much closer to him than Amy or I could get.

Seeing Paulie hooked up to all those tubes and wires for the first time, Amy, understandably, became totally unglued. Competing with a phalanx of tubes, wires, and all the other high-tech equipment a modern intensive care unit has to offer is not the idyllic picture a new mother has in her head when she envisions those sweet early bonding moments with her baby. I'm sure it just broke Amy's heart as she imagined the pain and discomfort Paulie must have felt when they were poking, probing, and hooking him up to all the equipment.

As helpful as it was to have a next-step plan of action for Paulie, the pace at which things were beginning to move was starting to hit me. This was no movie or television program where you could hit the pause button. This was all real, and it was happening to us, right now, ready or not. Finally, when an opening cleared around Paulie and I got a closer look, I could see that the paramedics had placed a small breathing tube into one of his tiny nostrils and an intravenous line into his arm. Along with the IV and the breathing tube, they'd also attached some kind of probe to Paulie's chest to monitor the movement of his heart and lungs.

Amy was now completely in tears. I tried my best to conjure up some method-acting bravado and transform myself into a confidence-inspiring in-control husband, not to mention the grizzled, unflappable journalist who has seen everything under the sun. Indeed, I had done several stories in and around hospitals, battlefield and otherwise, over the past several years. With one eye con-

stantly on the clock and the other on the script, I always knew how to shut it down emotionally in order to shoot the video or conduct an interview without becoming personally involved in the story. But now, seeing my own son in this fragile, helpless condition, my papier-maché facade instantly melted away and I, too, started losing it, just like Amy.

I so wanted to be the man—the stoic leader—for Amy at that moment, the smart, in control, resourceful guy who could figure this all out, save the day for my son, and bring a smile back to my wife's face. But it was all getting away from me, and I knew it. Despite my professional experiences and all my training, at that moment, I realized beneath it all, I was no longer the hotshot reporter with the great job and the A-list connections who could always get it together. I was just another terrified parent worried sick about his child. I was in no position to inspire Amy or anyone else at that particular moment. Breathing in and out and simply trying to survive to the next minute was about all I could manage.

Even with all the tubes and wires that prevented us from holding him, being reunited with Paulie there in the NICU was still pretty wonderful. Despite my sour attitude and lingering concerns about being blindsided with the news about Paulie's heart, I could clearly see with my own eyes that the Sibley nurses and the transport team knew what they were doing and were working well together. They also seemed as if they really cared about Paulie, which meant a lot.

Before long, however, another wave of anxiety swept over me as I thought about Paulie having to leave us for another hospital across town. I had just met this little

guy for the first time yesterday, and already I was experiencing the human magnet pull to be with him nonstop. I couldn't imagine what Amy was feeling or what her stress level was like as she watched the paramedics prepare to take Paul not only away from Sibley but farther away from her.

Being separated from Paulie while he was having tests done down the hall was tough enough. But Amy and Paulie had been physically connected for nine full months. All of his twists, turns, kicks, and anything else he had going on in there were shared experiences, the profound depths of which only she and Paulie could comprehend. And tonight would be the first time they would be apart after more than nine months together.

Although Children's was less than seven miles from Sibley, if those transport team paramedics actually were NASA engineers and they came over to tell us they were strapping Paulie on the top of a rocket for a trip to the moon, the emotional impact on Amy could not have been any worse. Seven miles or a quarter million, it was all the same for her. Her son was being taken from her and that was all that mattered.

The specific plan we came up with for the rest of the night was for Amy to stay at Sibley to continue recovering while I would go to Children's to be with Paulie. Thankfully, Amy's folks and her brother raced back to be with us. In between filling them in on the details of Paulie's heart condition, we decided Amy's dad would drive with me to Children's while her mom and brother would stay with her at Sibley.

Amy was still physically hurting, and as much as she wanted to ride with Paulie in the ambulance, she was in no condition to be racing through the streets of

D.C. to Children's or anywhere else for that matter. By now the paramedics had placed Paulie into a specialized, space-age-looking hard plastic bassinet contraption with openings for all the wires and tubes that needed to stay connected during the trip. As she stroked Paulie's tiny hand through the wires for the last time before they sealed up the plastic box around him, I could see Amy was devastated. The instant that ambulance door slammed shut, the God-sent infusion of sunshine that filled Amy's soul whenever she was near Paulie completely vanished.

The transport team leader had me sign the release forms so they could legally transfer Paulie, and then they were gone. Probably because of all the emotion and pain of seeing Paulie lifted into that ambulance, rationality went out the window, and Amy began to openly worry that something horrible might happen during the trip. Also, seeing them pull away with Paulie while I was still standing there beside her, Amy immediately started screaming at me to hurry up and follow the ambulance. Amy simply had to know that one of us was with Paulie, even if it was in a car trailing behind. Although a professional and highly trained medical transport team, operating at its highest level, was providing Paulie with the best care he could possibly receive, for Amy and her fragile state of mind the entire operation must have seemed just a few clicks away from a kidnapping.

Since I was totally clueless about what part of town they were taking Paulie to, the Sibley nurses quickly came up with a map for me so I could find Children's in case we lost sight of the ambulance. Amy's mother and her brother J.P. tried to comfort her as Big Paul and I rushed to the parking lot to find my car. By the time

the two of us found my car and plopped into the seats, I was emotionally tapped out. Having Amy's dad along for the ride to help me think, let alone keep me from driving through stoplights, was helpful. It also gave me some time to decompress a little bit and talk things through with someone who had tons of experience in dealing with hospitals and doctors. A highly successful medical device manufacturer in Chicago, Paul Hills really knew his way around the medical world, and I was extremely glad to have him as a resource.

Not having our own flashing red lights or siren, I, of course, could not keep up with the ambulance, so when we arrived at Children's, Paulie was already up in the Cardiac Intensive Care Unit on the hospital's second floor. I checked in at the Visitors Desk, and after we received our passes the front desk staff directed me to a side room where I had to fill out a bunch of medical forms so I could get Paulie officially admitted. After I was done with the paperwork, Paul and I headed straight for the elevators so we could get to the CICU and Paulie. When we arrived on the second floor, we checked in at the nurse's station, and I was immediately taken over to be with Paulie.

Children's CICU was a good-size open area with about twelve or fourteen beds separated by sliding curtains. Not much privacy for families visiting their children, but the configuration allowed the entire room to be monitored in one visual sweep from the nurses' station. I could see a few other parents huddled around their babies, but most of the sound in the room came from any number of high-tech monitoring and oxygen machines that whirred everywhere and constantly.

When I first approached Paulie's area in the CICU, a

couple of nurses were having a difficult time trying to locate the artery in his arm, which they needed to hook him up to his permanent IV. Finding an artery in a full-grown adult can sometimes be a challenge, so hitting an artery smaller than angel hair pasta must be a daunting task, even for a well-trained pediatric nurse.

Needle stick. Miss. Cry. Needle stick. Miss. Cry. Watching all this, I had one very specific thought: "Thank God Amy isn't around to see this." The most heartbreaking part was that it seemed as if each time they stuck Paulie's arm his cry got weaker, not the kind of tantrum you would expect from a healthy baby who was constantly being pricked with a needle. The entire episode probably didn't take longer than fifteen minutes, but to me and my worried-sick mind it seemed like hours. Obviously not able to be of assistance helping the nurses get an IV into Paulie's arm, I distracted myself by studying the machine monitoring all his vital signs.

Thankfully, the nurses eventually got Paulie's A-line in, so I took the opportunity to jump in to ask one of them to give me a quick tutorial on what all the monitor readings meant.

"Which one of these numbers do I need to worry about the most?" I asked.

I knew I was probably being a nuisance, but I simply had to know how everything worked. I needed to know the significance of every beep and buzz the machines made. The numbers. The ranges. I needed to know everything there was to know. Patiently, one of the nurses went through everything that was going on with Paulie and the machines he was hooked up to. If it wasn't for the fact that my one-day-old son was lying there hooked up, you might have thought I was producing a medical

documentary or preparing for a live shot on the latest in pediatric cardiology.

I am sure my behavior was an emotional dodge on one level, caused by all the pent-up insecurity of knowing I had zero control over anything that was going on. But somehow I believed if I could ask just the right, journalistic question or make a brilliant observation everyone else in the room had missed, I might be able to help my son. Even with an entire medical unit filled with highly trained doctors and nurses, if I was vigilant enough maybe I would catch Paul's numbers declining at the precise moment they began to drop and save the day. Turn this thing around.

Breaths per minute. Heartbeats. Oxygen in the blood. Blood pressure. My eyes were in constant motion darting from one set of numbers to the next.

If I could just figure out which one of the readings was most critical, I might be in a better position to do something to help my son. I am sure the nurses had me pegged as a high-maintenance type who was going to be a problem for them, but I simply had to be involved in some way—*any way*.

Talking with the nurse assigned to Paulie, I learned that because his heart was not pumping in the correct direction, he was having an extremely difficult time getting oxygen to flow from his lungs to his heart. I decided to concentrate on the oxygen level reading on the monitor. When Paulie's oxygen level started to dip, that would be a warning sign that he was about to go into a decline. From that moment forward I had a death-match, no-blink staring contest with the numbers on Paul's oxygen level gauge.

After about an hour of monitoring the monitor, I left

Paulie's side so I could call Amy at Sibley to see how she was doing. I didn't have the heart to tell her about the difficulty they had finding his artery. I also didn't tell her what I had learned about the oxygen levels in Paulie's blood. Amy was worrying enough for both of us, and I didn't think I had to share every minute detail I had learned while standing guard at my command post, especially now that I was officially part of the medical team minus the scrubs and a stethoscope. All Amy needed to know was that Paul was being well cared for—and he was.

After a little prodding I discovered Amy was holding out on me, too.

Since Paulie and I were both gone, she decided to check out of Sibley. I really discouraged Amy from coming to Children's. After much discussion I was able to prevail upon her to let her mother and brother take her back home so she could rest and get a good night's sleep. Tomorrow was going to be a huge day for us because we would be having an early-morning meeting with Dr. Martin to discuss specific options for Paulie following the results of some overnight tests.

In reality, despite my self-anointed bedside vigil, there was nothing either of us could do for Paulie that night, and we both needed to be clearheaded for the morning meeting with Dr. Martin. I told Amy I would come home to be with her, and we would go together to Children's the first thing in the morning.

"First thing?" she asked.

Not as much a question as it was a nonnegotiable clause in a lawyered-up contract, I replied, "Yes, first thing."

Deal cut; Amy was on board. After checking in on

Paulie one last time, Big Paul and I headed for the car so we could meet up with everyone else back at the condo.

As Paul Hills and I drove toward Georgetown, I silently reflected on the day's events and everything Amy and I had experienced over the past fifteen hours. I had never been to Children's National Medical Center until that night, and as I continued driving I realized I had gotten a little lost. Even though Children's is not that far from the U.S. Capitol or even the D.C. bureau of Fox News, it was in a section of the city I seldom visited. It took me a little while to find an identifiable street so I could get oriented and headed in the right direction toward home.

I chuckled to myself, thinking, even with all the heartache and mind-smashing pressure the day had brought, that I was still worried about embarrassing myself in front of my father-in-law by getting lost in my hometown. I mean, after all, I had lived in Washington for six years now; I should know these streets like the back of my hand.

But given everything we had been through that day, I could have probably driven in circles for the next hour and a half and I don't think Big Paul would have noticed—or cared if he did. We were both drained and eager to change the topic to anything other than doctors and hospitals, if even for a few minutes. Needing a cathartic release, Big Paul and I talked about whatever popped into our heads.

With me still searching for a familiar street to drive down, Paul turned to me and said, "How about a see-through when we get back?"

"You bet. Belvedere on the rocks for me!" I responded. Belvedere vodka, that is.

Back in Paul and Barbie Hill's upscale Barrington Hills neighborhood outside Chicago, "see-through" is a slang phrase for any cocktail someone can literally see through, usually a clear liquor drink, straight or on the rocks. More times than not, a martini. One of Big Paul's friends back home employed the phrase frequently, and we had joked about it often, adopting it as our own shorthand code.

I was happy to be talking about anything other than heart disease, if even for a short while. With the two of us laughing and conspiring about something as silly as our see-throughs, I realized how negative and sad I had been all day. As I continued to talk with Paul, I was reminded that Amy has some of his best qualities, not least of which are her drive and determination. Reflecting on Amy's obsessive need to get to Paulie in Sibley's NICU earlier in the day, I remembered an encounter she'd had just a few weeks before when we went to see a movie not far from our condo in Georgetown.

I should say, of all the beautiful inner and outer qualities Amy possesses, she is an amazingly strong, disciplined, hardworking, straightforward, bold, and honest person. She also has a heart of gold and is incredibly generous, just like Big Paul and her entire family. But, I should add, Amy is also a very security conscious, streetwise, city girl from Chicago, who is wicked smart and very aware of her surroundings. She is not about to let anyone con her, walk over her, or rip her off in any way.

After we watched our movie, Amy went into the restroom at the theater and encountered a homeless woman who was washing her hands. Upon seeing Amy in her extremely pregnant state, the woman smiled and said, "So, you're going to have a boy?" A little thrown,

Amy smiled back and said, "Yes, how did you know that?" The woman proceeded to give Amy a hug and said, "That's my gift, honey." The woman went on to whisper to Amy, "I just want you to know there is going to be something very special about your son. I don't know exactly what it is, but he is going to be very, very special."

Amy hugged the woman back and she immediately came out to me in the theater lobby. Not having her purse, Amy asked me if I had any cash on me. I reached into my pocket for a twenty-dollar bill, and Amy went back into the restroom and gave it to the woman she had been speaking to.

Later, telling me about the encounter, Amy said for some reason she felt a strong spiritual connection to the woman, almost like they had met somewhere before. I had forgotten all about the homeless woman until now. That woman was right. Master's champion or not, God had, indeed, blessed us with a very special child. And even though his journey on this planet, however long or short, was starting out rough, if Paulie somehow survived the challenges confronting him, surely he would be equipped to handle just about anything else life ever tossed his way.

A chance encounter with a homeless woman who knew how to coax a twenty-dollar bill from a gullible participant? An angel sent down from heaven to tip us off about what was to come? I have no idea. I have even less of an idea if God still sends angels down to earth to help us out of scrapes of one kind or another. But I am continually amazed how certain people—winged or otherwise—sometimes seem to appear in our lives at precisely the moment we need them there.

Reflecting on Amy's encounter with that woman, I immediately thought about the circumstances that first brought Nurse Beth Kennedy into our hospital room. The fickle finger of fate? The luck of the draw with the Sibley nursing schedule? A well-trained nurse who took her job extremely seriously? Divinely sent by God? I had no idea how Beth Kennedy came into our lives. In many ways it didn't matter. I thanked God for her, whatever her mode of transportation. In fact, earlier in the day, Amy and I both started referring to Beth as Our Angel for her persistence in trying to figure out why Paulie's color was off.

Throughout that meeting in our room with Dr. Martin, the entire time I was thinking we needed to have an expert come in and give us a second opinion on Paulie's condition. We were just being hit with too much life-and-death medical information at once, especially from a random, on-call doctor who happened to respond to a page while driving to a completely different hospital on a different case.

What I didn't realize at the time was that Dr. Martin was not just a random on-call doctor who happened to be driving past Sibley responding to a page. He was a world-recognized cardiologist who headed up the Cardiology Department at Children's National Medical Center, the very place where Paul was now being cared for. Dr. Martin's particular expertise is performing echocardiograms, diagnosing pediatric heart disease, and teaching other doctors how to do the same. He was one of the best people in the world we could have been talking to about Paulie's situation, and we didn't even know it.

Thinking back about the day, I realized how fortunate

we were that our new nurse *happened* to notice Paulie's color the first time she saw him, and one of the world's top cardiologists *happened* to be driving past Sibley at the precise moment the page went out.

I knew deep down it was going to take something altogether different than a few see-throughs to help us cope with what we would be facing in the days ahead. But even though the gathering clouds looked scary and dark, I got the sense we might not be taking this journey alone. There just might be someone looking out for us—helping us to see our way through the storm.

CHAPTER FIVE

One Day Closer

Amy and I had a fitful night. I got two hours' sleep at most, and I know Amy got even less. In the middle of the night I woke up, turned toward Amy's side of the bed, and saw she was gone. Down the hall, the rhythmic sounds of the breast pump machine were coming from Paulie's room. How sad Amy must have felt at that moment. She was so looking forward to having Paulie home with her: feeding him, doting on him, snuggling with him, and all the other things a first-time mother dreams about doing with her new baby. Now, in the middle of the night, Amy was sitting alone in the dark, in the very room and the very chair in which she was supposed to be nursing Paulie—and he wasn't there.

Amy and I spent a lot of time getting that room all fixed up and just right for Paulie's arrival: multicolored art on the walls, a black wood crib with leopard print pillows, a pullout couch, and a big white stuffed tiger we had already nicknamed Simba. The best thing of all was a comfortable white glider rocking chair we thought would be great for coaxing Paulie back to sleep in the

middle of the night. It was just the perfect nest of a room for Mom and Dad to spend quality bonding time with the newest addition to the family. Now Amy was sitting in that room all alone.

Before we fell asleep, Amy told me she cried all the way home from Sibley. With her brother J.P. driving Amy's car and her mother up front, Amy sat in back next to Paulie's empty car seat. Amy had been dreaming of that special moment when all three Baiers would be leaving Sibley together—me driving and she loving on Paulie all the way home in that backseat. She played that iconic coming-home-with-baby scene a thousand times over in her head. Wanting that first trip home from the hospital to be absolutely perfect, Amy even went to the local fire station to make sure the car seat was properly installed. Riding through the streets of Washington next to that car seat without Paulie in it really got to her.

After we got home, Amy took a hot shower. Still crying, and with the water rushing against her head, Amy told me it was almost as if she could hear Paulie crying all the way back at Children's National Medical Center. We held each other very close that night, both of us sobbing at various times. It's funny how that would happen. When Amy was having a particularly rough moment, I somehow seemed to have just enough in my emotional tank to comfort her. And when I started to hit bottom, Amy had something for me: a hug, a pat on the back, or just the right word of encouragement to preempt any impending spell of darkness that was trying to descend.

Despite feeling heartbroken about being back home without our son, whenever Amy was breast pumping, even with tears in her eyes, I could still see a glimmer of that old Amy Hills Baier spirit trying to shine through.

Amy had read several articles about breast milk and how wonderful all the natural nutrients were for new babies. Now that Paulie was in a fight for his life, Amy had her game face on and she was on the job.

By keeping up with pumping, freezing the milk, and storing it, Amy was committed to doing everything in her power to get Paulie as strong as she possibly could. We really didn't know specifics yet about what he was facing surgically, but Amy was totally convinced if she was faithful with her breast pumping every four hours, she would be having a direct impact on Paulie's chances for survival.

Apart from all the natural nutrients and vitamins she would be supplying Paulie, on a whole other level it gave Amy something specific she could do, a project to help her stay positive and not succumb to any dark moments brought on by worrying about the unknown. Amy is extremely organized, and I noticed she had already marked the refrigerator calendar with her round-the-clock "feeding times" for Paulie. She also cleared out an entire section of the freezer and prelabeled several empty plastic milk pouches with dates and times for pumping. Every four hours, no matter how tired or stressed, Amy would be up and pumping milk.

The nurses at Children's assured me they had pumping equipment and a small private room there in the CICU whenever Amy needed to use it. Even though she was probably going to spend most of her days and nights at Children's, Amy would be able to keep up with her project—her new life mission, really—to get Paulie as healthy as possible and ready for his surgery.

Throughout Amy's pregnancy, and even more so when we got closer to her delivery date, all my buddies

with children were constantly busting me out about how my life was going to drastically change once I became a dad. They razzed me about how I would be joining them in the Sleep Deprivation Club. Soon, they told me, I would be living the life of a zombie and waking up all hours of the night to change diapers, heat bottles, and rock my little guy back to sleep—all while I was completely dead on my feet.

After a night of complete sleeplessness, they assured me, I would stumble into work the next day totally exhausted but exhilarated and amazed at how productive I could still be on the job. In a perverse way, I was really looking forward to joining that club. I wanted in and I wanted all the merit badges. It was a rite of passage.

Although my friends had unique stories about the births of their own children, to a man they all warned me: "Don't leave the hospital any earlier than you have to; you'll be home soon enough—then you won't be getting any sleep at all!" Here I was; I wanted to stay another night with Paulie at Sibley, but because of his transfer to Children's, Amy and I were forced to come home earlier than we wanted.

In a sense, I had been awarded my membership badge in the Sleep Deprivation Club with an asterisk. Now I wasn't getting any sleep because Paulie *wasn't* home with us. It was ironic. I wanted all the worst-case scenarios my new baby would assuredly bless me with: screaming in the middle of the night, changing nasty diapers, cleaning up vomit. I wanted it all.

But there were no dirty diapers, no cries in the middle of the night. No 3:30 a.m. negotiations with Amy over whose turn it was to get up and deal with a screaming baby. Instead, I was lying in bed wide awake, listening to

my sobbing wife down the hall, and worried sick about my one-day-old son who was hooked up to wires and tubes in a strange hospital across town.

With Amy done with her breast pumping and back down for a few minutes' sleep before we had to get up and go to Children's, I quietly slipped out of bed and made my way into the kitchen. It was early on Sunday morning, and I went out front to grab the *Washington Post*. As I reached for the paper I could see headlines about a jeep rigged with explosives slamming into Glasgow Airport, a new universal health care bill going into effect in Massachusetts, the role of Independents in the 2008 presidential race, and an article about former president Bill Clinton joining his wife, Hillary, for their first joint campaign appearance in Iowa.

I was normally up to my eyeballs with news 24/7, but as I unfolded the paper it occurred to me that from the moment we drove to Sibley Thursday night until now, I had pretty much checked out from everything else going on in the world. Aliens could have landed on the National Mall to deliver a galaxy-tested interstellar plan for balancing the budget and I wouldn't have known a thing about it unless one of the nurses happened to mention it to me in passing on my way to the hospital cafeteria.

The Washington news clock starts anew each week with the Sunday morning news and public affairs shows—*Fox News Sunday*, NBC's *Meet the Press*, ABC's *This Week*, *Face the Nation* on CBS, CNN's *State of the Union*, and C-SPAN's *Washington Journal*. I had been so out of it newswise I had no idea who the guests were on my own network's Sunday show, let alone any of the others.

Even though I was clueless about what news stories had transpired over the past two and half days, to be perfectly candid I wasn't totally unplugged. For better or worse, I still had my Blackberry with me the entire time I was at Sibley and Children's. For a while there, before the wave of smartphones hit the shores of D.C., it seemed as if everyone in town working in politics or the news business had a Blackberry—or, as they were jokingly called because of their addictive nature, a Crackberry.

So while I was on the job checking Paul's monitor readings at Children's the night before, like Amy, I had come up with my own special project. Feeling powerless in my efforts to help my son, the only thing I could think to do was scroll through the names in my Blackberry contact list to see if I knew someone—*anyone*—who might know something about Children's, its cardiology department, pediatric heart disease, or anything else that might help me get a better grip on things.

I was already thinking, as any parent would, if Paulie's case was as serious as Dr. Martin said, I wanted him in the best pediatric heart hospital in the country. Through several e-mail exchanges with one friend, I found out he knew a doctor at Children's who might be willing to talk to me. This doctor knew the inner workings of Children's cardiology department and told my friend that Dr. Martin was the real deal—"nobody better," he said.

In the meantime, I received several e-mail responses from friends who had been working on a Best Hospital project for me. The notes I received all seemed to repeat the same three hospitals as being among the best in the country for complex cases like Paulie's: Children's

Hospital in Philadelphia, Children's Hospital in Boston, and Children's National Medical Center here in Washington, where Paul currently was.

One friend told me Children's in Washington had one of the best, if not *the* best, pediatric heart surgeons in the world for extremely complicated cases such as Paulie's: Dr. Richard Jonas. I am sure Dr. Martin mentioned Dr. Jonas to us at Sibley, but I was so discombobulated by everything we were being hit with at the time, I was having an extremely difficult time holding on to information.

After I got back home from the hospital late Saturday night, I received a call from the doctor who worked at Children's. He told me Dr. Jonas used to be at Children's Hospital in Boston and had been recruited to D.C. just a few years before. He said when Dr. Jonas was still in Boston, Children's sent their trickiest heart cases to him up there. He was that good and that well respected. It was apparently quite a coup for Children's National Medical Center when they were able to recruit Richard Jonas to join their cardiology department.

As with any news story I ever covered, it was a luxury to have someone on the inside to bounce things off of. Happy to have this doctor as a source right there at Children's, I asked him if I could stay in touch over the next several days as I received more detailed information about Paulie's situation. "Sometimes I get the feeling you doctors hold back and don't always share exactly what is on your minds, especially when asked specific questions about how things might turn out," I said. My new doctor-friend-source assured me I could call him anytime if I was getting frustrated and felt my questions about Paulie's case weren't being answered.

Before we knew Paulie had any medical issues, I'd sent out an e-mail to family and friends announcing the new addition to our family. Over the past two days, I'd received several notes of congratulations, encouragement, and welcome into the Holy Order of the First-Time Parent. Now, as word started getting out that Paulie was in trouble, I received a whole new wave of notes from concerned family members and friends asking what they could do to help.

To a person, they all said they would be praying for Paulie, Amy, and me and thinking good, positive thoughts. While Amy was sleeping for a few minutes before we headed out the door, I hopped on my laptop and wrote a group message so my family, friends, and colleagues at Fox would have a better idea about what was going on:

July 1, 2007, 6:56 AM, Sunday
Subject: Not as we expected…

Thank you all for your kind words and good wishes after the last e-mail. Now we'd like to ask you for something else—your prayers. After almost a full day with Paul and after he got a completely clean bill of health, Paul started having a hard time breathing. After multiple tests, doctors told us he has congenital heart disease that requires emergency surgery.

There are basically a few things wrong with his heart and the major arteries around it that need to be fixed. Fortunately, doctors caught it in time and he has been transferred to Children's National Medical Center, one of the best hospitals in the world for this kind of treatment. Paul

is in the Cardiac Intensive Care Unit and will have to have surgery in the next day or so.

It's a tough time, but we are a family of fighters, and we know he's going to pull through. We would really love it if everyone could say a prayer for our little guy—we really believe that can work. We know he can be a modern-day medical miracle. This isn't what we expected, but it's what we are dealing with. Thank you all for your support through this difficult time.

Bret and Amy

Once Amy woke up, she reminded me that her father wanted us to join him, J.P., and Amy's mother for breakfast at their hotel before we all drove together to Children's. Amy might have been my wife, but she was still Big Paul's little girl, and he wanted to make sure she started off the day—and what surely was going to be a very difficult week—well fed.

Paul Hills is your classic get-it-done, no-obstacle-too-big, world-changing type A personality kind of guy, and one of the most successful businessmen I have ever met. No doubt feeling every bit as powerless about Paulie's situation as I did, Big Paul probably thought if he could at least get us all together and fed he was doing something practical to help us get focused and ready for our meeting with Dr. Martin and his team later in the morning.

Amy and I had only been married for two and a half years, but by now I think I had her quirks, mannerisms, and idiosyncrasies pretty much nailed. All through breakfast, I could see she was about to jump out of her

skin, she wanted to be with Paulie so badly. It wasn't long before Amy started instructing each of us to hurry up and finish eating so we could get out the door and on the road to Children's. Amy simply had to get to her son.

The second we got our visitor passes at Children's, Amy was off and running for the CICU and Paul. It wasn't as though she was nervous or even crying at that point. It was more basic—more physiological—than that. Amy was simply going to burst if she didn't get to Paulie. Other than mothers who have carried a baby, I doubt any of us can really understand what she must have been feeling at that moment after being separated from her newborn son for the past twelve hours.

When we arrived at the nurses' station at the CICU, we were told only two people could be at Paulie's bedside at a time. Amy and I went in while the rest of the family camped in the small waiting room just outside. Amy let out a sigh of relief when she saw Paulie. Immediately, her entire countenance lightened as if someone had clicked a switch inside her. She was a completely different person; Amy Hills Baier was back.

The way they had Paul hooked up to the monitors and breathing tube, Amy wasn't able to hold him, so she had to settle for rubbing his skin and talking to him. Despite not being able to snuggle with him like she really wanted to, Amy seemed to find a measure of peace just being with Paulie. I could sense her stress level begin to drop the instant she started stroking his soft skin and nuzzling her face against his. It was something to see. Paulie was the extreme critical care patient, but if I didn't know better, I would say he was having some sort of healing effect on Amy.

Along with storing up breast milk, Amy was also convinced Paulie would do much better in the hospital the more he was spoken to and physically touched—talking to him, singing to him, stroking his hand, and holding him in the chair next to his bed whenever we could figure out how to get those wires and tubes sorted out.

I believed the same things about therapeutic touching, talking, and singing to Paulie as Amy did, but she seemed to know it all so instinctively, deeply, and with fervor. It was as if Amy had been training for this role her entire life. In fact, with her family already in town, my mother coming, and more brothers and a sister-in-law on the way, Amy was already concocting a plan whereby Paulie would have a family member with him—"loving on him," as she put it—pretty much around the clock. Since the two grandmothers, Barbara "Barbie" Hills and my mother, Pat Baier, would surely be performing the heaviest lifting, Amy had already started working up schedules for what quickly became known as the Grandma Brigade.

While Amy was continuing to love on Paulie as much as she could through the wires, having already appointed myself a member of the official medical team the night before, I checked in with the *other* staff to see about Paulie's overnight numbers. Before long, Dr. Martin came into the CICU, reintroduced himself to Amy and me, and asked if we could meet with him and a few members of his cardiology team in a side conference room. Amy immediately ordered me to go to the waiting room to get her mother and father so the next shift of family love could clock in at Paulie's bedside while we were in our meeting.

With Dr. Martin was another cardiologist, Dr. De-

neen Heath, and Dr. David Stockwell, who headed up the CICU. As it turned out, Dr. Stockwell was my secret source from the previous night's phone call. In many ways I felt like I had an ace in the hole—someone I could talk to off the record and on the side if I needed help cutting through the medical jargon and hospital legalese.

By now, I was fully aware Dr. Martin wasn't just a random doctor who had responded to the page from the Sibley nurses yesterday afternoon. He was chief of cardiology at Children's and codirector of Children's Heart Institute, and by the way everyone on the floor was treating him I could clearly see he was *the man*. With his calm demeanor and very caring tone, as Dr. Martin began to speak I felt a tinge of guilt for spending so much time checking him out on the Web and with my investigative team of D.C. friends.

"As I told you yesterday over at Sibley, Paul has some very significant heart issues, so it may take a little while to explain this all to you. So let me start at the beginning," Dr. Martin said.

Holding hands, Amy and I looked into each other's eyes, silently telling one another we loved each other. After a sleepless night, we both did our best to focus on every word Dr. Martin spoke during what surely was going to be the most important meeting of our lives.

Dr. Martin said that usually when he is called into a situation like he was yesterday at Sibley, there are basically two kinds of congenital heart disease he is looking for: noncritical and critical.

"With noncritical heart disease, if it is discovered before the baby goes home from the hospital, that's great. But if not, it's not going to harm the child. The problem

will present itself at some point in time and can be dealt with then: a little hole in the heart or a mild blockage. Whatever it is, it can normally be dealt with down the road," Dr. Martin said.

"But when you find critical heart disease, such as the type Paulie has, you must immediately set the wheels in motion," he said, explaining the activity of transporting Paulie to Children's the night before. Dr. Martin told us that before he performed an ultrasound of the heart or echocardiogram at Sibley, he had determined a fair amount by simply listening through a stethoscope and physically placing his fingers on Paulie's chest wall just above his heart—the precordium.

One of Paulie's heartbeats, the prominent impulse, was way too strong, Dr. Martin explained. That immediately told him that one of Paulie's heart chambers was working at too high a pressure and was totally unsustainable. Continuing to listen through the stethoscope, Dr. Martin discovered that along with one chamber working too hard, Paul's heart sounds were abnormal. He said he could hear that Paulie was missing one of the sounds to his outflow. Dr. Martin drew us a picture to illustrate what he was talking about.

"In a normal heart that is working the way it's supposed to, you typically hear a *lub-dub* sound," Dr. Martin said. "That second *dub* sound—if you listen closely enough—is actually two separate sounds," he explained. "It's actually a lub-*dub-it*," he said.

Listening to Paulie's heart, Dr. Martin said he could hear that it was missing the second part of the dub-*it*. "Typically when that second '*it*' sound is missing, it means one of three things: the blood vessel is missing altogether, it is blocked, or it's in the wrong loca-

tion," he said. Everything Dr. Martin learned up to that point, he said, was done basically by touching Paulie's chest with his fingers and listening through the stethoscope.

Next, Dr. Martin got a more detailed look at Paulie's heart by performing an imaging test, or echocardiogram. It wasn't long before he knew exactly what was going on. "I discovered that with Paulie it was a combination of not only that blood vessel being in the wrong location, but also being much smaller than normal," Dr. Martin said. The technical description of what was going on with Paulie's heart was "transposition of the great arteries" and something called a "double outlet right ventricle," Dr. Martin told us. He said the artery that should be going to Paul's lung was the one that was actually leading to his heart, and the artery going to his heart was the one that should be going to his lung. "Paulie's blood is flowing entirely in the wrong direction," Dr. Martin said.

It was nearly impossible to visualize, let alone comprehend what Dr. Martin was telling us. Although I was scared to death, I was also completely amazed that Paulie's heart had somehow figured out how to reroute itself for survival. Along with those arteries performing the wrong functions, Dr. Martin said they were also both on the same side of the heart—the right side. Paulie would have to have surgery so they could perform something called an arterial switch to get the arteries back to their proper positions and doing what they were originally intended to do.

In addition to all that, Dr. Martin explained that Paulie had a few other things going on. "Along with the arteries being in the wrong place, they are also much

smaller than they should be," he said. The technical condition is called pulmonary stenosis. Basically, the artery was pinched to the point where blood was not flowing properly.

Dr. Martin said Paulie also had something called aortic stenosis, where the aorta is smaller than it should be and makes it very difficult for blood to flow anywhere, let alone to those arteries that were in the wrong place and performing the wrong functions. The blockage in the aorta was also preventing blood from pumping to Paulie's legs.

Finally, Dr. Martin said Paulie had two holes in his heart, what he called a VSD and an ASD. He explained that the holes—if that was all that was going on—would not be that big a deal. But in combination with everything else going on in there, they, too, presented a real problem.

With all those things laid out for us, I was amazed Paulie was actually still here with us. The fact he was alive seemed to indicate, to my untrained eye anyway, that his heart decided to call an audible, improvise, and do whatever it had to do to survive until somebody could come along to fix it.

Having heard all the complexities going on with Paulie's heart, I was still dumbfounded that at least some of this wasn't discovered during any of Amy's sonograms or checkups, especially since Dr. Martin could basically figure this all out within sixty seconds by using his fingers and a stethoscope. Restraining myself from playing the blame game, all I really wanted to know from Dr. Martin at that point was when could we get Paulie's heart fixed and who was going to do it.

Dr. Martin told us Children's was fortunate to have one

of the best surgeons in the world for the type of complicated surgery Paulie would need: Dr. Richard Jonas. He said Dr. Jonas performed more than 350 highly complex surgeries every year, and although Paulie's combination of issues put him on the extreme high end of the complexity scale, Dr. Martin said he was confident Dr. Jonas could figure out the best way to approach it. I told Dr. Martin we had already done some research on Dr. Jonas, and Amy and I had pretty much agreed he was the guy we wanted working on Paulie's heart.

Dr. Martin said his immediate concern with Paulie was something he described as "a ductal-dependant lesion," meaning Paulie's life was dependent on the blood vessels being maintained in the open position. If those blood vessels closed up, Paulie could go downhill very quickly, Dr. Martin explained. "The immediate name of the game is to sustain Paulie by keeping the vessels open while we continue running tests to make sure he doesn't have anything else going on," he said. Sustaining Paulie and keeping the blood vessels open was primarily the job of the drug PGE1, a prostaglandin that Dr. Martin had put Paulie on over at Sibley.

PGE1 is in many ways a miracle drug that ensures the blood vessels stay open so as to allow blood to bypass blocked or severely constricted arteries. Dr. Martin explained that when he went through his early medical training, PGE1 didn't exist. As a result, babies discovered with congenital heart disease in those days had to be operated on almost immediately and always with urgency and drama attached. Now, with PGE1, even though there are always exceptions, it's very rare that babies need to be operated on in the middle of the night, Dr. Martin said.

The real miracle of PGE1 is that it gives doctors time to conduct a proper assessment of the baby, looking at the whole child. They are not forced to jump right in and start cutting without having all the information surgeons need or would like to have. "Unfortunately," Dr. Martin said, "even though PGE1 allows us time to do more sophisticated testing, there are some potential side effects."

"What side effects?" I asked.

"For one, Paulie could stop breathing," Dr. Martin said.

Amy and I exchanged quick, worried glances. Dr. Martin explained this was the reason that monitoring Paulie's breathing, respirations, and blood pressure was so critical right now. Because the PGE1 was doing exactly what it was supposed to be doing, relaxing the blood vessels, Dr. Martin said that if Paulie's blood pressure dipped below a certain level, there could be a whole other issue of having to give him fluids to bring the pressure back. If the blood pressure dipped too low and stayed there for an extended period of time, it could also cause damage to the kidneys, he explained.

Dr. Martin said that while everyone, understandably, was focused on Paulie's heart right now, he didn't have the luxury of knowing that was the only thing causing him problems. He explained that in cases where babies have heart disease, typically 15 to 20 percent have other organ abnormalities in the brain, the kidney, the spine, or their lungs. "PGE1 allows us to keep Paulie in a safe, stable situation while also giving us time to do a better assessment of what else might be going on with him," he said. "Even though Paulie has a very, very serious heart condition and definitely needs surgery, he doesn't need it today or tomorrow," Dr. Martin said.

Seeing the dazed looked in our eyes, Dr. Martin seemed to instinctively understand our confusion. "I know this is hitting you hard and without warning, but congenital heart disease is actually the most common birth defect babies have, affecting one out of a hundred live births," he said. "The truth of the matter is, we have done a very poor job telling the world about heart disease. So most folks, like yourselves, are not prepared for it when they hear it," Dr. Martin said.

Truer words have never been spoken.

Dr. Martin continued to explain that because of the PGE1, whenever Paulie did go into the operating room, he would be completely stabilized and in a much better position to survive the trauma of surgery on his small body. I asked how long, realistically, Paulie could be sustained the way he was on PGE1. Dr. Martin said if he didn't take a turn for the worse, Paulie could probably be sustained in his current condition for ten days to two weeks.

"What if Paul does take a bad turn? Will he immediately be taken in for surgery?" I asked.

The only problem, Dr. Martin said, was that Dr. Jonas happened to be out of the country right now and wouldn't be back in Washington for another week. I looked over at Amy, and by the look in her eyes I could see she was crushed. After all the stellar information we had received about Dr. Jonas over the past twelve hours, my gut told me Paulie was probably exactly where he needed to be, and Dr. Jonas was the best guy to operate on him. Dr. Martin said Paulie was currently stable, and he thought they could keep him in that condition until Dr. Jonas returned. In the meantime, he said, they would be sharing images of Paulie's heart with Dr. Jonas

while he was out of town so he would be fully briefed upon his return.

Dr. Martin said that although they pretty much knew everything going on with Paulie's heart, the only remaining question to be answered was the specific approach Dr. Jonas would take to fix it. He said he really wouldn't know details on that until Dr. Jonas returned and they could sit down and discuss it. Dr. Martin said one of the things you get with Dr. Jonas is his ability to improvise and be creative. "Once he gets in there, if something pops up that was not altogether clear in the echocardiograms, there's no one better than Richard Jonas to figure it out," Dr. Martin said.

Apart from all the immediate medical questions I was asking, Amy wanted to know about the kind of life Paulie would have after the upcoming surgery. "Will Paulie's surgery be a one-time fix, or will he need more?" she asked. "Is there a chance he might need a heart transplant down the road? Would Paulie be able to play sports? Will Paulie be able to run around and hang with the other kids in school? Will he be able to play soccer with the other kids?"

Drs. Martin, Heath, and Stockwell were all very professional and caring as we hit them with our barrage of questions. But after a while it became like some sort of awkward chorus. Every time we asked a variation of our "Will Paulie be able to..." question, what we would hear back was "Don't know," "Can't really say," "Hard to say," "No guarantees on that."

Amy and I had dozens of more questions about the overall situation and about Paulie's future, but my overriding specific question had to do with the clock. Would Paulie be able to hang in there long enough for

Dr. Jonas to return, or were we taking too big a risk by not sending him somewhere else to have immediate surgery?

I asked twenty-seven different variations of that one question, but I could not extract a definitive answer. The doctors simply were not in a position, medically or legally, to offer us any guarantees or to tell us what we should do. At that moment, it became clear to me this was going to be our decision—and ours alone.

I asked if there was anyone else at Children's who was close to Dr. Jonas's level of expertise in performing the kind of surgery Paulie needed. Martin said there really wasn't, but if we didn't have a comfort level waiting for Dr. Jonas to return, we always had the option of flying Paulie to Boston or Philadelphia.

"Okay. Let's say we decide to wait for Dr. Jonas to come back, and then Paulie starts to decline. Will you be able to give us enough of a heads-up so we can get him on a helicopter to Philly or Boston?" I asked. Dr. Martin paused and then answered, "I think we will," but again, he gave no absolute guarantees.

As I thought more about the overall situation we found ourselves in, I got even angrier that Paulie's condition was not discovered during Amy's pregnancy. If we had been given any kind of advance notice on the baby's condition, maybe we could have figured out how to keep Dr. Jonas in the country in the first place or possibly had Amy's delivery date delayed through medication until he got back. A thousand scenarios were racing through my head, including whether Dr. Jonas could get on a plane and come back early from wherever he was.

I didn't care what it cost. If we could get Dr. Jonas

back earlier, I would happily pay his airfare. Even if we had to send a private plane to pick him up, we would figure that out, too. I would do anything I had to do to keep my son alive. Dr. Martin said he would check to see if Dr. Jonas could come back any sooner.

By this point, although I was truly appreciative of the doctors' time and their obvious concern for Paulie, I had grown increasingly frustrated about not getting specific answers to any number of questions we were asking. After several minutes, in a fit of stressed-out, righteous, indignant parental anger and desperation, I kicked into an entirely different nondeferential gear I suspect the doctors didn't think I had in me.

"Look, I know this is all legal, and you can't offer any guarantees. I get that. I am not going to sue anyone. Paulie is our only child. I just need to know one thing. If he were *your* son, what would you do? Would you send him to Boston or Philadelphia now, or would you wait for Dr. Jonas to get back?"

It was almost as if I was anchoring a news program with only a few seconds left on the clock and my politician guests had been tiptoeing through the tulips the entire show avoiding giving a direct answer on whether they were going to vote for or against a controversial piece of legislation. To a person, every one of the doctors in this medical lightning round answered, "Wait for Jonas." "Wait for Jonas." "Wait for Jonas."

Finally! I found the magic key to the mystery lock so I could get the advice we desperately needed. Given the lawyered-up country in which we live, I was thinking this kind of scene probably plays out every day in every hospital in America: doctors knowing what kind of advice they would like to give parents but not feeling free

to give it because they put their hospitals and themselves in legal jeopardy if they are too specific and things don't turn out.

Amy had gotten very quiet during the later half of the meeting, and I worried that the positive vibe she had from being around Paulie had drained out of her, especially after hearing the scary specifics of what was going on with Paulie's heart. The fact that we were in the middle of a giant guessing game about Paulie surviving until Dr. Jonas returned didn't help, either. Amy seemed intensely worried and started to get this vacant look in her eyes.

Telling the doctors we needed to discuss this by ourselves, Amy and I thanked them for their time and we headed back to Paulie's bedside. As soon as we arrived in the CICU there was a commotion going on around Paulie. His A-line had come out again, and the nurses were struggling to get it back in. I had seen the identical thing the night before, but this was Amy's first time, and she really started to freak out.

Watching all this unfold, Amy started questioning why it was taking so long to get the line back in and why the nurses were "hurting" Paulie. The nurses, understandably, asked us to temporarily leave Paulie's bedside so they could fix the line without all the nervousness and second-guessing. So Amy and I left the CICU and went to the waiting room to be with her parents. While there, we filled everyone in on the meeting with the doctors.

When I got to the part where I explained that Dr. Jonas was overseas, I could see Big Paul was about to blow a gasket. He immediately told me to find out where he could send a private plane so we could get

Jonas back. I told him they were already looking into that for us. After a while, I checked back with Dr. Martin and he informed me Dr. Jonas could not come back early because he was giving some very important lectures that couldn't be canceled, and he was also doing some volunteer work with Project Hope in Asia.

Amy once told me her father had a favorite expression he often used throughout his career in business: "If you have a problem that can't be solved with money, then you have a really serious problem," he would say. Getting Dr. Jonas back to operate on Paulie was apparently not a money issue, so by Big Paul's calculations this was a really serious problem.

Growing up, Amy was extremely close to her father. He was always the fixer, the man who could solve any problem that came down the pike. But like the rest of us, Paul Hills couldn't really do a single thing that was going to change the equation for Paulie. Feeling every bit as frustrated as we were, Big Paul was having a very tough time trying to figure out what he could do to help. After all, his daughter might very well lose her first child. And while Paulie was my first son, he was also Big Paul's first grandson, not to mention his namesake.

Still bothered by the scene at Paulie's bedside with the IV, Amy was extremely agitated. We were all there in the waiting room openly talking about whether Paulie would be able to hang in there long enough for Dr. Jonas to return or whether it would be better to fly him to Boston or Philadelphia for immediate surgery. In the middle of all this family frustration and stress, Big Paul blurted out, "In my sixty-one years of life, this is the worst thing I have ever experienced!"

Suddenly, in the middle of this bona fide American

family meltdown, I looked over and saw a nurse rushing our way. I thought there must have been some kind of emergency down the hall she was running to deal with. To my shock and horror, I suddenly saw where the nurse was going. Amy had collapsed right there in the CICU waiting room and fallen into a clump on the floor.

Immediately, the nurse called for help and a gurney. A medical team arrived to take her to the emergency room down on the first floor. With Amy now on the gurney and being rolled down the hall, I held her hand as I ran alongside. The paramedics put an oxygen mask on Amy's face. Although she was not unconscious, Amy was definitely dazed and confused about everything that was happening.

Once we were in the emergency room, a team of doctors descended on Amy and started checking all her vital signs. They immediately put her on an IV so they could get some fluids in her. I told the doctors Amy had just given birth and was under a lot of stress with her baby being in the CICU. I also told them Amy didn't get any sleep the night before, was hypoglycemic, and had been breast pumping.

Amy was still out of it, but after a few minutes I could see she was breathing a little better. Soon her color started to return, and the doctors in the ER told me she was stabilized and not in any danger. After Amy was feeling better, the nurses in the ER gave her some graham crackers to munch on, and it was just Amy and me in a small curtained-off area in the ER. We were at rock bottom. The trauma of the A-line episode had really gotten to Amy, as did hearing all the specifics about Paulie's heart. Since we were getting no sleep and

were totally stressed out, it was clear to me we needed to change some things if we were ever going to be in a position to help our son.

With Amy lying there in the ER, the oldest patient at Children's National Medical Center, I somehow found the strength and clarity I had been lacking over the past twenty-four hours.

"Okay, Amy. We've obviously been dealt a tricky hand here. But we need to change our focus, or none of us is going to make it out of here. We have to put blinders on. From now on, this is just about Paulie, and *only* about Paulie. We need to figure out what is best for him and not worry about anything else. We need to get back to basics. We are his parents, and we need to make some tough decisions," I said.

"I think we need to wait for Dr. Jonas to come back. He is the best there is, and we just have to hope and pray—and trust the doctors—that Paulie will get stronger every day he is here. No Philly. No Boston. He's staying here," I said.

By the look in her eyes I could tell Amy was with me.

"We also have to take care of ourselves, otherwise we won't be of any use to Paulie. We have to eat. We have to sleep. And we have to trust each other. God gave us Paulie. But we are the parents God gave to Paulie, too. We can do this. We both need to buck up and not blame anybody for this. We need to trust God and trust the doctors."

I could see Amy was now listening intently, and a smile started to come to her face. I was now on a roll. "If Paulie is anything like his mom and dad, I know he will be fighting with everything he has. We need to fight *for* him here in this hospital the same way he is fighting

for himself. Let's put him in the best position we can to help him survive this," I said.

Having gotten all that off my chest, Amy and I were now both in tears. But these were not the tears of victims, worrying about all the unknowns, who dropped the ball, or who was trying to ruin our lives. Knowing we had turned an important corner, these were the tears of strength and release. We had our plan, and we both knew what we needed to do.

"One final thing," I said. "We are getting Paulie baptized right here in the CICU this week. I'll feel a lot better once we get Paul up on God's scoreboard."

Amy laughed, and at that moment, for the first time, I started to believe we were that much closer to getting Paulie out of there. After giving Amy a hug and a kiss, I said, "We're one day closer to taking Paulie home." Then, right there in that emergency room, behind those closed curtains, with screaming babies all around us, the oldest patient in the ER at Children's National Medical Center and I started a tradition we would continue till the day we were finally able to bring our son home: we gave each other a high five.

I called for the nurse to come unhook Amy's IV line. She had a little boy she needed to be with. And I had to find Dr. Martin and the rest of the family to tell them what the plan was.

"One day closer," I told Amy.

"One day closer," Amy replied. "One day closer."

CHAPTER SIX

Things Unseen

In the days immediately following our turnaround moment in the Children's emergency room, Amy and I became downright evangelical in our newfound mission—our decision—to transform ourselves into the two most positive, upbeat people on the planet. Not because we necessarily felt like it, but we genuinely believed being positive and uplifting would have a direct impact on Paulie's ability to fight and survive.

I was done with all the self-pity and the crushing waterfall of victimization I had allowed myself to get sucked under by constantly questioning who dropped the ball in missing Paulie's heart disease during Amy's pregnancy. What was done was done. That was all in the past.

Amy and I turned a serious psychological corner during her brief stint as the oldest patient at Children's National Medical Center. The blinders were now officially on. From now on this was strictly about Paulie's health, well-being, and future—nothing else. This was no longer about our personal hopes and dreams being

dashed. Not about what doctor didn't diagnose what or when. Not about blaming God for dealing us a bad hand. Like it or not, this was exactly what God had given us to deal with, so we were on the job.

Paulie needed us to be focused and forward-thinking if we were going to be part of the solution to help him get through this. The last thing he needed was negativity, second-guessing, or bickering by well-intentioned but openly worrying parents or family members. The residue of stressed-out parents and families always rubs off on children, no matter how old they are or whether or not they are in intensive care units.

Even though he was just two days old, after our self-directed halftime pep talk in Children's ER, Amy and I were committed to constructing a sort of protective shield around Paulie there in the CICU. We not only wanted him to have every spiritual advantage possible, we wanted everyone who came in contact with him—caregivers and stressed-out family members alike—to be infused with that same positive vibe, too.

We might not be able to control the intricacies of his complex heart, the numbers bouncing around on the monitors, or Dr. Jonas's travel schedule, but we could control our conversation, attitudes, and the overall atmosphere we created around Paulie's bedside. By eliminating any hint things might turn out badly, we wanted our son to know deep down in his two-day-old spirit that his parents were optimistic, had their winning game faces on, and were on the job for him. We owed him that much.

Whenever we were by Paulie's bedside or with family members in the waiting room just outside, we were constantly talking about that happy day when we—*all three*

Baiers—would finally be able to check out of Children's and drive home together. I might still be getting lost navigating the narrow streets between Children's and Georgetown, but as long as Paulie was in his firehouse-approved car seat and Amy was happily doting on him in the back, I didn't care if that trip home took all day. Visualizing and openly conversing about that day became our new mantra, inspirational thought of the day, and total obsession all rolled into one. We didn't know exactly how or when, but it *was* going to happen.

There is a scene in the film *Apollo 13* where longtime Flight Director Gene Kranz, played by Ed Harris, exhorts his engineers to do the impossible and bring astronauts Jim Lovell, Fred Haise, and Jack Swigert back to Earth after an oxygen tank explosion forces them to abort their mission to the moon. With the astronauts caught halfway between Earth and the moon in a dying spacecraft, Kranz, as played by Harris, bellows to a roomful of engineers and scientists gathered at Houston's Mission Control: "Failure is not an option!"

Later, hearing a colleague suggest the mission might yet turn out to be the worst disaster in the history of the U.S. space program, Kranz replies, "With all due respect, sir, I believe this is going to be our finest hour." That's the kind of attitude Amy and I wanted to have, especially when we were around Paulie. Despite the scary unknowns he was facing surgerywise, we, too, wanted this to be our finest hour.

Some days Amy and I were truly hopeful things would work out. Other times I am sure we were simply playacting our way through deep doubts, surreptitiously trying to convince each other things would turn out just fine. In many ways, it didn't really matter how we ar-

rived at the emotional or spiritual place we needed to be as long as we got there.

We knew of course that Paulie was hanging by a thread and could take a bad turn at any moment. But even though we sometimes didn't see how things could possibly turn out in his favor, Amy and I had just enough faith to believe the hopes and dreams we had for our precious son would one day come to pass.

I have always been a student in the "see it—believe it—achieve it" school of armchair philosophy. I tried my best to fill my mind with images of Paulie walking with me on the seventeenth fairway at Congressional as I spilled over with all my fatherly wisdom about girls, cars, school, and life—not to mention the best way to make par on eighteen. Deep down I knew I could very well be setting myself up for a big fall if things took a turn for the worse. But I desperately needed to change the channel in my mind and visually get Paulie out of that hospital bed, off the tubes and wires, and into his little-boy body at least six or seven years down the road.

On really good days I would see Paulie all grown up, going to high school dances, playing soccer, walking the links with me on a cool summer morning, and asking me if he should use the five or the six iron. Those were not just fanciful images or Jedi mind tricks I came up with so I could temporarily transport my brain out of the hospital. I regularly prayed for the day when those things—and a lot more just like them—would come to pass.

Occasionally, in order to catch a quiet moment away from the constant beeps and buzzes of the CICU, Amy and I would venture to a little chapel in the hospital where we would pray or sometimes just sit together and

hold hands. We enjoyed walking down the hall and into that chapel whenever we could, especially if someone in the family wanted some personal time with Paulie, or Amy and I needed somewhere quiet to sit and talk other than the waiting room or the coffee shop.

Dimly lit, with just a few plastic chairs scattered around, the chapel was not fancy, but it always had a warm and calming effect on us whenever we had the opportunity to slip in there for a few minutes. In the corner of the chapel stood a wooden stand holding a large Bible with a lace place holder for marking specific pages and verses. There was also a small stack of writing paper next to the Bible. I suppose the paper was there for folks to jot down verses, prayers, or other thoughts that might come to them during their times of reflection.

I doubt they teach this in theological seminaries, but I would often go over to that Bible, shut my eyes, flip the pages, and place my index finger on a random verse just for fun to see where I would wind up. Once I went over to the Bible and it was already open to the New Testament book of Hebrews. Someone had scribbled "Chapter 11 verse 1" on a piece of paper lying nearby. I read the verse: "Faith is the assurance of things hoped for, the conviction of things not seen."

Even though there were plenty of reasons to believe the mountain Paulie was climbing might be too steep, the verse captured how Amy and I were trying to approach that week in the hospital. Naively or not, we chose to set our eyes on that unseen hope—*the assurance*—that Paulie would hang in there long enough and Dr. Jonas would figure out the perfect way to reconstruct his heart. We were also trusting and believing

the Lord would be holding our hands every step of the way.

Beyond hope and faith, I also believed there was a wild card or X factor at work—Paulie himself. Looking into his eyes, I could see he was doing everything in his power to fight his way through this and come out the other side. I am not sure I could get any of the doctors to concur with me on this, but given the severe defects he was born with and the way his heart was rerouting the blood flow through his arteries, I was fully convinced Paulie had his own unique set of survival skills the rest of us knew very little about. Apart from being in one of the world's top hospitals and having some incredibly skilled doctors and nurses caring for him, I sensed Paulie had something just as important going on. He was a fighter with a warrior spirit.

Along with our renewed spirits and commitment to staying positive, Amy and I also became extremely proactive for our little fighter in the hospital that week. We were constantly agitating—nicely—for everything we thought Paulie needed to help get him healthier and stronger for his upcoming surgery.

Just one day into his hospitalization, we had already successfully negotiated with the CICU nurses to get all those wires and tubes extended a few feet so Amy could sit in the chair next to Paulie's bed and hold him to her heart's content. This wasn't simply about Amy feeling more like a real mom by being able to snuggle and rock with her son. We both believed the more Amy and other family members could hold Paulie, the more loved he would feel. Subsequently, he would be more secure, grow stronger, and ultimately be much better equipped spiritually and physically to deal with the highly invasive

nature of surgery, let alone surgery on his six-pound twelve-ounce infant body with a heart the size of a walnut and arteries smaller than angel hair pasta.

One day after our ER epiphany, Amy and I also followed through on our decision to have Paulie baptized in the CICU. Despite our relatively high spirits and renewed commitment to being positive and upbeat, we weren't kidding ourselves; we knew Paulie's life was on the line. We had intended to have him baptized in our local church by our parish priest when we got him back home to Georgetown, but given the sobering reality that there were no guarantees and the fact that Dr. Jonas wouldn't be back for another week, I felt strongly about having Paulie baptized sooner rather than later.

I know people of faith in various denominations have differing views on the meaning or significance of baptism, especially when it comes to babies and children. But for Catholics like Amy and me, baptism is a very important sacrament and long-standing tradition of the Church I wanted my son to be a part of. In the Catholic faith, the sacrament of Baptism is often called the Door of the Church because it opens the door to the other sacraments. Given all the unknowns we were facing, we at least wanted Paulie inside that door.

To be perfectly honest, even though I am a Christian and believe in prayer, if I had stumbled upon a *National Geographic* in the waiting room with an article about the healing power of ancient Pacific island dances, just to cover my bases I am sure I would have been rolling up the rugs and trying to find some hand-carved log drums on craigslist. I simply wanted to get anything and everything working in Paulie's favor that I possibly could, points on God's scoreboard or not.

On Monday afternoon, we closed the curtains around Paulie's medical bay and squeezed in several family members for the baptism. The CICU nurses helped us contact a priest affiliated with the hospital who could come in and perform the ceremony with little advance notice. Just like our wire extension project, even Paulie's baptism required that we bend a few hospital rules to make it happen the way we wanted. Somehow it must have slipped my mind to inform the nurses exactly how many congregants would be in attendance. With the two-person-per-bedside rule still in effect, just like trout fishing up in the mountains, let's just say we were over the legal limit.

The priest who performed the ceremony was very calming and had an extremely soft voice with what I decided must have been a Kenyan accent.

Packed in and huddled around Paulie's bed, we were accompanied by an electronic chorus of beeps and buzzes from the monitors throughout the CICU. After he read a few passages from the Bible, the priest anointed Paulie's head with oil and holy water. Next, Amy and I both said a prayer. Wiping away a few tears, I prayed, "Dear Lord, thank you for all the blessings you have given us and the biggest of our lives, the birth of our son, Paul Francis. We now turn him over to your care for his upcoming surgery and the recovery that will follow. Please be with all of us gathered here and help us get through this challenging time. Lord, please give us strength. Amen."

Amy also prayed. "Lord, help us give Paulie all the love we can give him. Please help us to prepare him for surgery. And be with our family as we put Paulie in your hands."

The priest then led the entire family in the Lord's Prayer. After a few closing remarks, the bedside ceremony was over as quickly as it had begun.

That baptism wouldn't exactly qualify as a high church ceremony. But because of where we were, the sardine-can closeness of family members huddled all around, and the fervor in our hearts as we prayed, that bedside ceremony couldn't have been any more meaningful if we had been planning it for six months and held it in St. Peter's Basilica in Rome.

Immediately after the baptism, Big Paul and J.P. had to leave so they could get back to their jobs in Chicago, while Amy's mother and rock, Barbie Hills, hunkered down for the long haul. Barbie, who always seemed to have a smile on her face, was there for her baby, and now her baby's baby. My mother, Pat Baier, had flown in from Florida and was also there to help us from the beginning of our time at Children's.

Growing up, my mom played a huge role in my life, and like Barbie with Amy, I am sure it must have been heartbreaking for her to see her child suffering as his own first child was holding on for dear life. Both Barbie and Pat were, once again, moms to their children, helping in any and every way they possibly could, always with smiles and tons of encouragement along the way.

Because Amy and I would typically stay in the CICU until ten or eleven at night, one of the grandmas would normally take the early morning shift with Paulie, arriving at Children's sometimes as early as 6:00 a.m. After our stop at the Starbucks near our condo, Amy and I would arrive at Children's a little later, around 8:00 or 9:00 a.m. Around noontime, the grandma not pulling early morning duty would typically arrive at the hospi-

tal with lunch for everyone. If Amy or I needed a break to catch some dinner or go back to the condo to take a shower or change clothes, one of the Brigade would cover for us at Paulie's bedside while we were away.

Once we returned from dinner, we would cut members of the Brigade loose so they could get some rest. The cycle would begin all over again the next morning around 6:00 a.m. It was blue-collar shift work pure and simple, designed to fulfill Amy's desire to have a family member with Paulie during as many hours as possible.

Over the next several weeks at Children's, the Brigade was happy to welcome various other recruits who flew into town to report for duty. Amy's older brother, Tom, and his wife, Darby, flew in from Chicago. And Amy was completely thrilled when her twin brother, Dan, was able to visit all the way from Colorado. Being twins, Amy and Dan have a unique, unspoken bond I suppose only they can fully appreciate. Dan's a big, strong guy, and knowing how deeply connected they are, I have often thought that when Amy got mad at me for something, Dan was probably mad at me, too, all the way over in Colorado. That's how strong their bond is. It meant the world to Amy to be able to see Dan rocking with Paulie, wires and all, in the now familiar blue rocker next to the medical bassinet.

My younger brother, Tim, also came in from North Carolina. My only sibling, Tim had followed me into broadcasting and was working as the weekend sports anchor for *SportsNight* at News 14 Carolina in Charlotte, North Carolina. Tim was ecstatic when I first told him the news of Paulie's birth on Friday afternoon. One day later, on Saturday night, he was covering the U.S.

Women's Open at Pine Needles Golf Club in Southern Pines when I called to tell him about Paulie's heart complications.

Paulie was Tim's first nephew, and knowing my brother I am sure he was already thinking about all the great uncle-nephew trouble he would be able to get in when Paulie got a little older. The news about Paulie's heart condition hit Tim, who was preparing for a 10:00 p.m. live shot when I called, really hard. Through the phone line I could tell he was completely devastated. First thing Monday morning Tim hit the road and drove from North Carolina to be with us in D.C.

Along with having family members around for encouragement and moral support, it was extremely helpful to have extra sets of hands to hold Paulie, run errands for us, or do any number of things that needed to be done those first few weeks. Amy's MO was to always be one of the two *legal* people by Paulie's bedside. Unless she had to leave to pump milk or use the restroom, that is pretty much where she stayed day and night. Although I always had dibs on the second legal spot, I would trade off with other family members so they could cycle in and spend time with Paulie and Amy.

Amazingly, Amy's calmness and strength during those first days at Children's seemed to be directly related to the amount of time she spent with Paulie, whispering to him, softly singing to him, touching his skin, and, of course, holding him. Amy found an incredible amount of joy and peace just being by his side. At a few days old, Paulie obviously wasn't saying much to us by way of encouragement or thanks for being there with him. But somehow, through his resilient spirit and sheer force of will, it was almost as if he was running the whole show,

sending out his own positive vibes to keep the rest of us energized, upbeat, and on the job.

Paulie's healing effect on Amy was real and not just romantic, touchy-feely mother-baby stuff, either. The more she could physically be with Paulie, the healthier, more energized—even less tired—she seemed to be. It was almost as if Paulie had some kind of secret energy source Amy had tapped into. With Amy emotionally and spiritually healthier by simply being near Paulie, the effect rubbed off on me as well. Paulie was keeping Amy calm. Amy was keeping me calm. And that, in turn, helped us keep the atmosphere—our protective shield—around Paulie hopeful and upbeat.

Let's face it: that first week at Children's was one gigantic family-style stress test. But with Paulie doing his job keeping his mother peaceful, even joyous, it not only affected the way Amy and I were interacting with each other, it allowed us to get out of our own heads once in a while and even reach out to the caregivers who were helping us and some other parents with their own children in the CICU.

Along with all the practical and emotional support we got from our families that week, Amy and I also received a ton of e-mails from concerned family members who couldn't be there with us, friends, and my coworkers at Fox.

Amy truly appreciated the prayers and good thoughts coming our way from across the country, but she was in such a special zone nurturing Paulie, she left it up to me to handle all the electronic communications, incoming and outgoing. Almost as though she was lying low in a high-tech spy movie, Amy was completely off the communications grid that week. The rest of the world was

simply going to have to wait a few weeks before she decided to log back in.

I, however, was a completely different case. Whenever I was away from Paulie's bedside I was reading and responding to the steady stream of good wishes and prayers filling my Blackberry in-box at a now constant rate. When word started getting out about Paulie's heart condition, that steady stream quickly developed into a gusher.

After sending out my group mail early Sunday morning before we first left for Children's, I must have received three hundred e-mail responses from coworkers at Fox, people I grew up with, schoolmates from Marist and DePauw, professional colleagues, and various other folks I had met over the years. I also received many special notes from several of my competitors/friends at the Pentagon and the White House: Jack McWethy of ABC, Jim Miklaszewski of NBC, and Jamie McIntyre of CNN, to name a few.

I am not sure how it happened, but we even received an e-mail from a priest at the Vatican who said he was praying for us. Whether divinely inspired, a Kevin Bacon *Six Degrees of Separation*, or simply the daily miracles of the Internet doing what it does best, I truly believed all those positive messages and thoughts were having an effect.

After sending out my Sunday morning e-mail message, one of the first responses I received was from my former Fox News colleague and White House press secretary Tony Snow. Short and to the point like the succinct writer he was, Tony's note captured the spirit, tenor, and tone of hundreds I received during that first week at Children's:

July 1, 2007, 7:52 AM, Sunday
To: Bret Baier
Subject: Re: Not as we expected . . .

Prayers up, buddy. God bless.

Tony

That short, to-the-point message was especially meaningful because I knew Tony was not only a person of
faith, he was no stranger to hospitals and fears about the
unknown. Just two years earlier, while he was still anchoring *Fox News Sunday* on the Fox broadcast network,
Tony was diagnosed with cancer of the colon. His mother
had died of the same disease at the age of thirty-eight, so
Tony surely knew what he was up against.

But after six months of treatment, Tony's doctors told
him the cancer had gone into remission. Then in April
2006, Tony left the network to become chief spokesman
for President George W. Bush. After almost a year at the
White House, Tony's cancer returned and had spread to
his liver. Tony made the decision to undergo an intensive, aggressive chemo regimen that took him away from
the White House for more than a month.

After being away for five full weeks, and just two
months before Paulie was born, Tony returned to the
White House briefing room to robust and heartfelt ap-
plause from all the gathered reporters, including me. It was
an incredibly powerful day to be in that briefing room.
Despite all the huge news moments that have occurred
there over the years, the day Tony returned is one I will
never forget. Network news reporters, producers, cam-
eramen, radio broadcasters, and veteran newspaper and

wire reporters alike were all moved by Tony's triumphant return and the amazing spirit and courage he displayed.

"Not everybody will survive cancer, but on the other hand, you have got to realize you've got the gift of life. So make the most of it," Tony said.

He went on to talk about the roles faith and prayer were playing in his battle. "Anybody who does not believe that thoughts and prayers make a difference, they're just wrong," he proclaimed. "I won't tell you how it's going to work out, because I don't know. But we obviously feel optimistic. And faith, hope, and love are a big part of all of it."

Tony also told everyone in the room that if they ever found themselves in similar circumstances to make sure they didn't try to go it alone: "The support I've received from you and from my colleagues at the White House and people around the country has been an enormous source of strength. There's no way to quantify it, but you feel it. You feel it in your heart. And in many ways, that may be the most important organ for recovery. To have the kind of spirit and to realize that, in my case, I'm unbelievably lucky and unbelievably blessed—and really happy to be back."

Caught up in that special moment with all my colleagues, I am sure some of Tony's insights washed over me that day. Now, just two short months later, and on the receiving end of similarly intentioned good wishes and prayers, I knew exactly what he was talking about. As distraught as Amy and I were about the overall situation with Paulie, surely our newfound energy and good spirits were not all self-generated simply because we willed ourselves to be positive. It was much deeper than that. In many ways during that first week at Children's,

I sensed we were being carried along and cushioned by support provided by those who were praying for us.

It's one thing to say "I'm praying for you" to simply and honestly offer encouragement to those facing particular challenges so they know they are not alone in their fight. However, in light of Tony's joyous example and the way he was handling his cancer with an almost otherworldly spirit and grace, I was convinced the prayers and good thoughts on our behalf were making a difference. As Tony said, there was no way to quantify or measure their power.

Fully aware that our Paulie had life-threatening heart disease, there is no way to explain the peace, joy, and calmness Amy and I had in our hearts during much of that time of turmoil and heartache. On a purely human level it made no sense at all. There's no other way to explain it other than the pure grace of God and all those folks who had been praying for us.

Even as I write this it is difficult to accurately describe being on the receiving end of the prayers and positive thoughts people were sending our way during those days. One particular e-mail I received really got my attention, especially later when I had time to reflect on its full meaning and specific timing. The note came from my mom's brother, Jim Savard, a retired professional pilot living in Colorado.

July 1, 2007, 2:11 PM, Sunday
Subject: GOD—FAITH . . .
To: Bret Baier

Dear Amy, Bret, and Paul,

Paul, today at 10:54 Mountain Time over 2,500 folks said a

prayer for you. The folks were attending the 10:30 service at Cherry Hills Community Church in Highlands Ranch, Colorado. The passage today concentrated on the Book of Daniel, and specifically on the fact that our success is in the Hands of God and we must have Faith.

Amy, Bret, and little Paul—HAVE FAITH! God Bless!

Warmest regards,
Jim Savard

Very spiritually minded, Jim took my early Sunday morning request for prayer to heart, and just a few hours later he shared it with members of his local church in Colorado. About the same time Jim's church was praying for us, two thousand miles to the east, the Baier-Hills clan was in the midst of its all-American family meltdown in the CICU waiting room.

After Amy's collapse and our trip to the Children's emergency room, we were at emotional rock bottom. Amy and I both felt lost and alone, in a 2007 version of our own modern-day lion's den. Safe to say, at that precise moment I wasn't feeling superconfident God was down there in that ER with us. Then, suddenly, as if someone reached down, flipped a switch, and gave us an infusion of energy and clarity, Amy and I made our "one day closer" pact and our decision to be positive and forward-thinking.

Right then and there in that ER we decided we were going to trust the doctors, trust God, stop being victims, wait for Dr. Jonas to get back, and be part of Paulie's solution. It was a true moment of renewal and rebirth for us. At our lowest point, that turnaround episode came

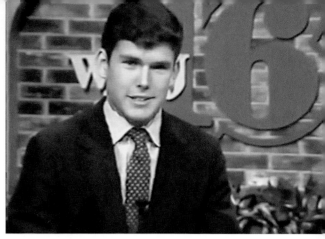

My early days working at WJWJ-TV in Hilton Head, South Carolina—1992. For the record—the *16* on the building is not a reference to how old I looked when I first started appearing on air.

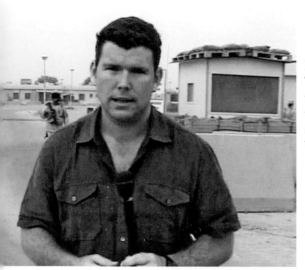

Reporting in Baghdad, Iraq—2003. This was during one of twenty-three trips I made to the region while working as Fox News national security correspondent and chief White House correspondent.

Reporting on Taliban attacks outside Kabul, Afghanistan—2005. Meeting many of the men and women who serve our country in extremely difficult circumstances convinced me *The Greatest Generation* should not be reserved only for heroes of the past.

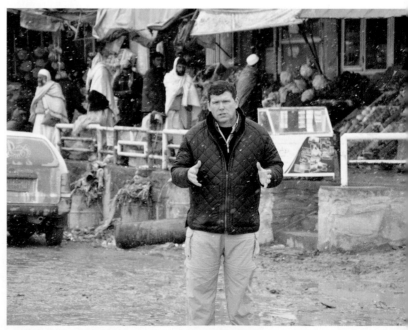

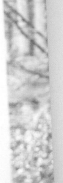
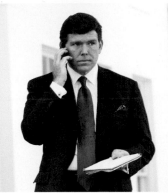

Working the phone outside the West Wing as chief White House correspondent — 2007. Despite the challenges of the job, I never lost my sense of awe and wonder about where I went to work each day.

Airborne news conference with Defense Secretary Donald Rumsfeld aboard Air Force Three. That's me in the lower right corner preparing to unfurl a question that hopefully might generate some news.

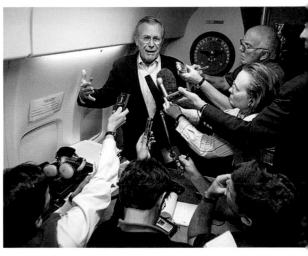

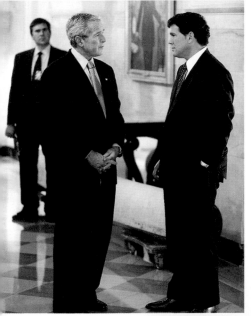

Shooting some informal hallway walking video with President George W. Bush following a sit-down interview in the White House Map Room — 2006.

Interviewing President Barack Obama in the Blue Room just three days before Congress passed his signature health care bill, the Affordable Care Act, also known as *Obamacare* — March 2010.

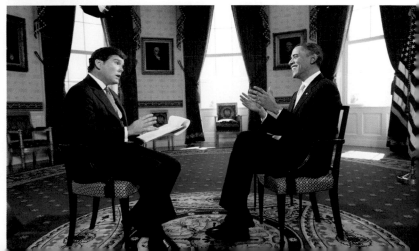

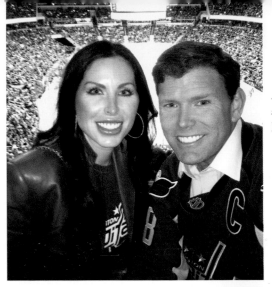

Amy and I enjoy a night out at a Washington Capitals hockey game.

Amy and I attend the Children's Ball charity event in Washington, D.C. I think I forgot to send Amy the memo about maximum height for high heels.

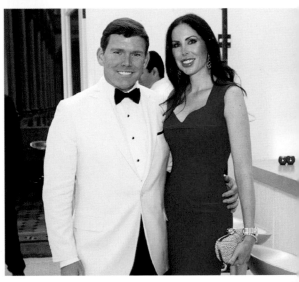

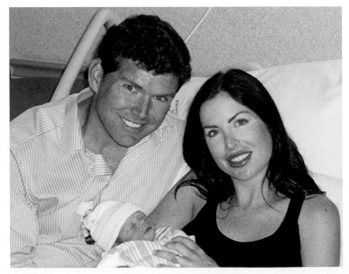

Happy times in the Sibley Hospital maternity ward just a few hours before we learn that Paul was born with life-threatening congenital heart defects.

Despite serious heart complications, Amy and I still enjoy being able to do some of the normal things with our precious two-day-old Paul.

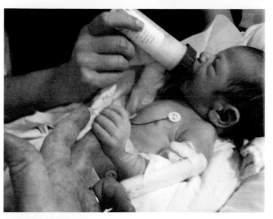

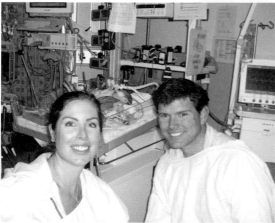

Amy and I are all smiles in the Children's Cardiac Intensive Care Unit (CICU) immediately following Paul's highly successful first open-heart surgery.

The Baier-Hills troops gather around Paul following his first surgery. Amy and I wouldn't have made it through any of Paul's hospitalizations without the loving support of our family and friends.

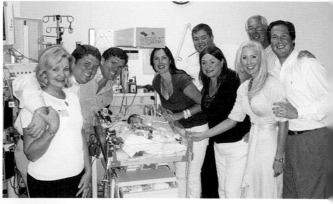

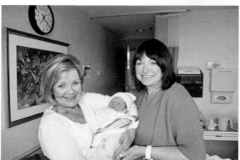

The legendary "Grandma Brigade"—our mothers, Pat Baier and Barbie Hills. Two loving moms once again stepping in to help their children—always with smiles and tons of encouragement.

Paul makes a new friend one day before returning to Children's National Medical Center for his second open-heart operation—2008.

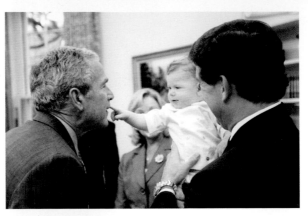

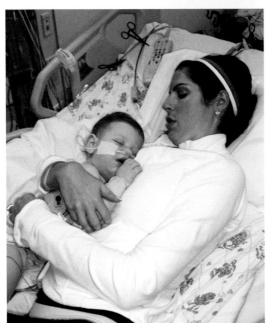

Amy snuggles with Paul in the Children's CICU a few days after his second open-heart surgery.

The doctors, nurses and staff at Children's National Medical Center have been there for us throughout all of Paul's hospitalizations. Amy and I were constantly amazed by their dedication, professionalism and the way they treated Paul as if he were one of their own.

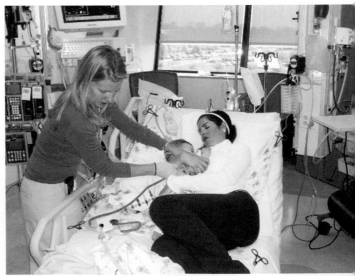

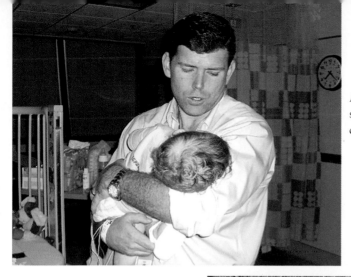

A few days after his second surgery, I do my best to coax Paul back to sleep.

Paul and I tend to serious matters at Congressional Country Club in Bethesda, Maryland. Many nights during Paul's first year I would lie awake and wonder if this picture would ever become a reality.

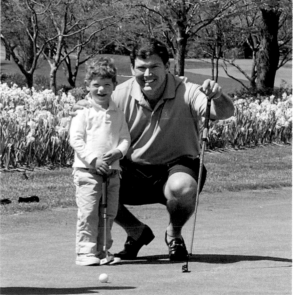

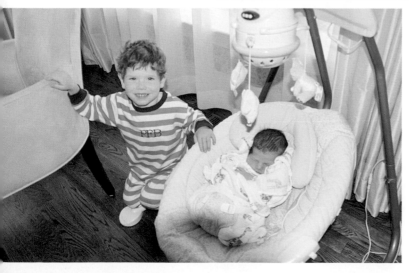

Paul welcomes his brand new brother Daniel to the world—July 2010. These days the boys are inseparable—best friends for life.

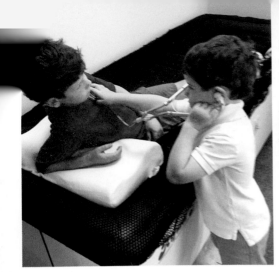

Dr. Daniel gives big brother Paul a medical check-up in Naples, Florida—August 2013.

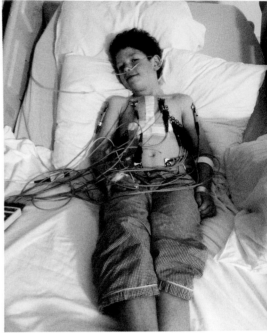

Smiles begin to return after Paul's third open-heart surgery at Children's National Medical Center—September 2013.

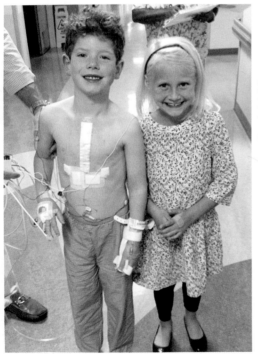

Paul walks the halls of Children's with his good friend Alice Caroline Marriott who reminds him "the more you walk, the faster you can go home."

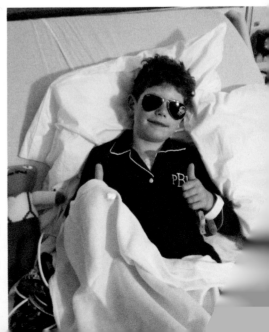

Cool Paul chilling out in recovery and eager to head home from the hospital. With all he has been through, I sometimes have to remind myself that Paul is still only six years old.

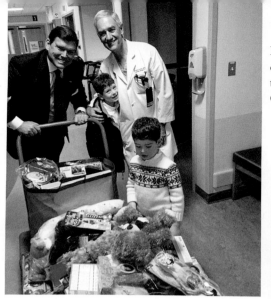

Paul, Daniel, Dr. Richard Jonas and I deliver Christmas presents to some of the kids on the heart and kidney floor at Children's National—December 2013.

All four of us decked out in running gear at the Race for Children 5K in Washington, D.C. just days after Paul's third open-heart surgery.

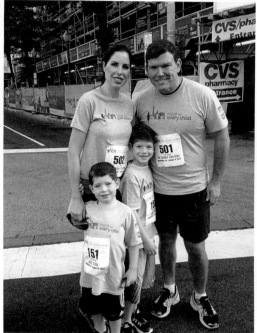

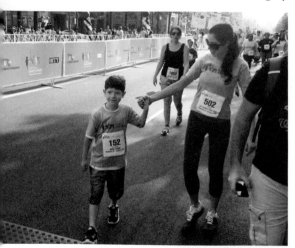

Paul crosses the finish line—a true champion in every sense of the word.

Amy, Paul and Daniel join me on the *Special Report* set in the Fox News Washington bureau. Regarding future jobs in television—Amy always gets a kick out of telling people all three of her boys have *Baier Hair.*

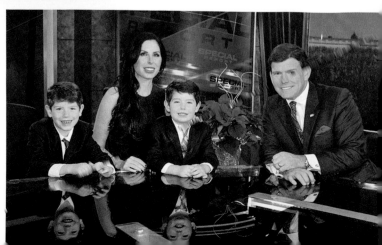

at just about the same moment Jim Savard and the other members of Community Church in Highlands Ranch, Colorado, prayed for us. The e-mail from Jim telling us about that morning prayer by 2,500 of his fellow worshippers landed in my in-box just as Amy and I returned to the CICU to tell Dr. Martin we made our decision to stay at Children's and would be waiting for Dr. Jonas to return instead of transporting Paulie to Philadelphia or Boston.

I received several similar messages from individuals and even a few other churches and synagogues that week. But Jim Savard's e-mail really got me thinking about the seriousness and efficacy of prayer, especially by people who truly believe in its power.

Another thing that really got to me that week at Children's was the way my colleagues at Fox News reached out to make sure I was okay. My bosses in the D.C. bureau and up in New York told me to take whatever time off I needed to deal with Paulie's hospitalization and surgery. My friend and mentor Brit Hume was a constant source of inspiration and encouragement to Amy and me, with a steady stream of phone calls, e-mails, prayers, and insights. Like Tony, Brit knew his way around grief and heartbreak. Brit's son Sandy, a rising star in the world of D.C. political journalism, had died ten years earlier at the age of twenty-eight. Whenever Brit talked to me about the grief Amy and I were feeling and about trusting God to carry us through, I knew he knew what he was talking about.

One of the most meaningful calls I received that week was from Fox News CEO Roger Ailes. I was not expecting the head of the entire company to reach out to Amy and me, but he did. Roger is known in

the media world as a take-no-prisoners, conquer-the-mountain kind of guy who took Fox News Channel from total obscurity in 1996 to the top of the cable news world in four short years. But what most people don't know about Roger is that beneath that tough guy media titan persona is a heart of gold. Roger, with no fanfare, has spent a lifetime reaching out to help people in and out of the media world who, for whatever reason, needed a break or some help to get back on their feet.

Another thing most people don't know about Roger is that throughout his childhood he was plagued by various medical problems. As a young boy, Roger was a hemophiliac. Growing up in the 1940s and '50s in the rough-and-tumble working-class town of Warren, Ohio, I am sure he had every opportunity to call it quits, but he didn't.

Once, as a preschooler, Roger bit his tongue and the bleeding was so bad he almost died. According to the recent biography *Roger Ailes: Off Camera*, by Zev Chafets, Roger's father, Bob Ailes, put him in the family car and raced to the Cleveland Clinic sixty miles north where they were able to stanch the bleeding and save Roger's life.

Throughout his childhood, Roger missed a lot of school due to any number of other mishaps that led to similar bleeding incidents. Once, a bicycle accident left him with serious internal bleeding. In her diary, Roger's grandmother calculated he had to have eighty-five separate injections in one three-week span. So Roger knew his way around hospitals and certainly had some special insights into what Amy and I were going through.

Seeing I had an incoming call on my cell phone from Fox headquarters in New York City, I quickly made my way to an area of Children's where I knew I could maintain a signal. Immediately, I recognized Roger's identifiable, no-nonsense, no-BS, midwestern, Joe Everyman cadence.

"How ya doin? You hangin' in there?

"Little tough, Roger, but we're hanging in there okay," I said.

"I can only imagine," Roger replied.

Then he added: "I don't want to take too much of your time. But I want you to know you have my full support. I also want you to know you can take as much time as you need to deal with this and be with your family. If you need anything at all from us—*from me*—just let me know."

Roger's long pause between "from us" to "*from me*" spoke volumes. He was not reading from a script or checking off an item from a Calls to Make Today list. This was heart to heart, not CEO to employee. I am not sure I knew Roger's history with hemophilia at the time, but he did allude to all the time he had spent in hospitals as a child when he said, "When Paulie survives all this, he is going to be one tough son of a gun."

Roger's remark made me laugh. His words about the qualities this episode was going to build into Paulie's character reminded me that I needed to be thinking down the road and far beyond the upcoming surgery.

After a week at Children's, I was getting to know my way around the place pretty well. Even though the exterior of the building looks like a spaceship zooming through the galaxy, every hallway you walk down reminds you that the people working there are single-

minded about their old-fashioned mission to help children in need. Children's has been all about that mission for more than 140 years now.

Five years after the end of the Civil War, in 1870, the entire Washington region was still devastated by the incredible loss of life on both sides—fathers, sons, brothers, and husbands. With poverty and hunger rampant, a group of doctors in the District decided to join together to do something about the most vulnerable victims of the times: poor sick children.

Thus, Children's Hospital of the District of Columbia was incorporated on December 5, 1870, operating out of a rented row house not far from where the Metro Center train station now stands. With the ongoing mission to help children in need, Children's arrived at its current location on Michigan Avenue in northwest Washington in 1977.

One thing you notice when you enter the hospital for the first time is how bright and colorful the place is. The front desk is in a natural-light atrium area with several multicolored hot air balloons hanging aloft and suggesting complete freedom and dream-filled flight. After several days there, I have to admit I had more than one whimsical thought that one of those balloons might be untethered for Amy, Paulie, and me so we could fly away to our own problem-free Emerald City, wherever those places are hiding.

Another thing you notice about Children's is the amazing range of socioeconomic, ethnic, and cultural, diversity represented. Regardless of political or religious inclinations, world views, or any of the other categories that typically divide us, the bridge-building, unifying dialogue of the realm at Children's is simply and purely

what's going on with your child and what's the plan for getting them well.

Since Amy was always by Paulie's side, I spent a lot more time than she did wandering the halls of Children's and camping in the small waiting room just outside the doors to the CICU. I had the wonderful opportunity to meet many other parents pulling the same kind of hallway-waiting room duty I was: waiting for surgeries, consulting with doctors, sharing background stories, exchanging heartfelt words of encouragement, laughing together, sometimes crying together, and always—*always*—talking about the day we would finally be able to get out of there.

On a fairly regular basis I had the opportunity to talk with a couple whose daughter, Maggie, had been in and out of Children's over the better part of the past year. Now nine months old, Maggie had been through a staggering nine separate surgeries since she was born. By the way her parents talked about her, you just knew Maggie had some serious spunk.

Whenever Amy would leave Paulie's bedside to go to the private room where she would breast pump, she would walk right by Maggie's bed and smile at her.

It was heartbreaking to see other parents during our time at Children's doing their best to be with their child as much as possible, but who because of jobs or distance couldn't be there as much as they wanted. It forced me to count my blessings that I had a job with extremely supportive bosses, plenty of family members to help us, and lived less than five miles away.

Dr. Richard Jonas was scheduled to return to D.C. on Monday, July 9, and Dr. Martin thought Paulie's surgery would probably be scheduled a few days after

that—probably Thursday, July 12. I knew the PGE1 Paulie was on was essential for sustaining him till his surgery, but I couldn't get out of my mind the possibility that too much of the drug, over an extended period of time, could cause him to stop breathing.

Assuming Paulie's numbers didn't drop into the danger zone, we were told that upon his return Dr. Jonas would be performing several easier surgeries before he got to Paulie's. First hearing this, I was a little confused, but eventually it made complete sense. Because Paulie's case was extremely complex, and given the fact that Dr. Jonas does two, sometimes three, highly complicated surgeries every day, he wanted the extra time to think through the best approach to take with Paulie.

Once back in town, Dr. Jonas needed two to three days to prepare by looking at various images of Paulie's heart, meeting with the sonographers, and consulting with the team of cardiologists who had been putting their heads together on the particular nuances and intricacies of Paulie's case.

The remainder of the week waiting for Dr. Jonas to return was a blur of activity as we performed all the rituals of going to Children's every day. Starbucks run in the morning, relieving the early morning shift of the Grandma Brigade, Amy breast-pumping every four hours, breaks for food in the hospital cafeteria, checking Paulie's monitor numbers, interacting with nurses and doctors, triple-checking Dr. Jonas's schedule, late night trips home to Georgetown, Amy breast-pumping at the condo, middle-of-the-night phone calls to Children's to check in with the overnight nursing shift, waking up, then repeating the process with our morning stop at Starbucks.

During our drive every morning from our condo to Children's, I would typically make a left turn on 16th Street not too far from the White House. Whenever I made that turn I would see the reflection of the White House in my rearview mirror. To be perfectly honest, I didn't know if I should take that as a cruel reminder of how our lives had been completely turned upside down or a sign of hope that one day soon some normalcy might return and I could get back to work. In either case, given the seriousness of Paulie's day-to-day battle and the upcoming surgery, every day when I made that turn I had my daily reality check that there are things much more important in this life than money in the bank account, careers, status, or where you happen to work.

Every time we told folks at Children's we were waiting for Dr. Jonas to return to perform Paulie's open-heart surgery, their eyes always opened big and wide and they would brighten up as if you had just told them the Messiah was returning. It was eerie; no one had anything bad to say about the guy. By the reverence everyone showed when we spoke about him, when Dr. Jonas finally did return to town I half expected him to enter the city limits by walking across the Potomac.

As nervous as we were approaching Paulie's operation, with each day Amy and I also got more and more excited about finally being able to meet the man we were now convinced would be saving our son's life. Personally, I didn't care if Dr. Jonas walked across the Potomac, parachuted in with the Golden Knights, or got the one-dollar Bolt bus special out of New York City, as long as he got here soon.

Friday, July 6, was a big day for us at Children's: Paulie's one-week birthday. Amy and I were extremely

grateful to God for giving us our son and keeping him strong for the week. We were also incredibly thankful to our family and friends for their support through some very difficult days.

July 6, 2007, 10:46 AM, Friday
Subject: A thank-you—and an update

First of all—thank you for all of your support and all of your prayers. We have really been uplifted knowing that so many people have been thinking about or praying for us. Here's the update: Paul's surgery is now tentatively set for Thursday morning, the 12th.

One reason it has been pushed back is because he has been doing very well and is gaining strength—he's stable, he's eating, and we are holding him about as much as any baby can be held. The other reason is to give arguably the best surgeon in the world for this type of surgery, Dr. Richard Jonas, time to analyze things after being out of the country for 10 days.

We feel we are in very good hands and feel very fortunate that we are able to hold Paul, talk to him, read to him, feed him, and show him love during this time. (When he's with me, he learns a lot about golf.)

Paul has a combination of things wrong with his heart—but the overall diagnosis is called double outlet right ventricle with transposition.

Basically, that means that the two main arteries going to and coming from the heart are in only one side of his heart

(the right side) AND in addition to that they are doing the wrong jobs. They're switched, taking blood to the body or taking blood to the lungs. One of the arteries is bigger than the other because it was being used more, which also creates a problem. Also, he has a hole in his heart (which is how he's moved blood around now)—as well as a blockage in his aorta that brings blood to his legs.

It sounds overwhelming—I know—but Dr. Jonas has seen similar cases, and while it's very complex, he has successfully completed this surgery before. Many families with children who have been through complex heart surgeries have emailed or called us to show us that more and more success stories are happening every day with how far this surgery has come.

So we're optimistic.

While we feel amazingly blessed to be able to spend this time with Paul, it's also been very tough to wait for surgery. As you can imagine, we have good days and bad days—the emotional roller-coaster is on a constant loop. But as the days go by we feel stronger (in large part because of the support from all of you!). Family members from all over the country have been coming in to meet Paul and help out. So we're hanging in there.

Paul was baptized in the hospital this week. Almost all of our family was there for an emotional ceremony in the Cardiac Intensive Care Unit. We know the week ahead is going to be very challenging—so we welcome any thoughts or prayers as we head into surgery on Thursday. We really have been comforted by them this past week.

As a new father and a husband, I never knew that I could feel this much love for our little baby who is now going through so much so soon—and for my wife, who is showing amazing strength just days after giving birth.

At 12:34 p.m. today, Paul will be one week old.

Today, we are one day closer to bringing him home to us—and that's how we have been approaching each day. We feel very blessed to have Paulie with us to begin with, and one day we'll look at the scar on his chest and consider it the most beautiful thing in the world.

Thank you again for your support.

Bret and Amy

As I hit the send button on the mail, I was thinking, hoping, and praying that next Friday I would be sending another message telling everyone Paulie had come through his open-heart operation with flying colors.

"The assurance of things hoped for," I thought. "The conviction of things unseen."

CHAPTER SEVEN

Special Hands

"Bret, this is President George Bush calling. I know you and Amy are standing by Paul's side as you prepare for his surgery tomorrow. And I just wanted to let you know that I am praying that all goes well. Hang in there, buddy. Put your faith in the doctors, and I know you'll put your faith in God."

I couldn't believe I had just missed a personal phone call from the president of the United States and let it go directly to voice mail. Of course, I didn't know it was the president calling when I decided not to take the call. Looking down at my phone, I knew it was probably an important Washington mover or shaker of one kind or another because all it said was 202, nothing else.

But let's face it, there are many important, not to mention self-important, people in D.C. That call could have been from just about anyone in town: a congressional press secretary trying to "clarify" remarks his boss shouldn't have made in an e-mail that shouldn't have been sent, or a political consultant wanting his senator client's name mentioned in every VP short-list story

Fox did between now and the 2032 presidential election. You get the picture.

The exact moment my phone rang Amy and I were standing outside a small coffee shop at Children's National Medical Center talking with *truly* one of the most important people in our lives, the head of the cardiology department and codirector of the hospital's Heart Institute, Dr. Gerard Martin. Dr. Martin and his cardiology team had been taking care of Paulie for the past twelve days in the Children's Cardiac Intensive Care Unit, and Amy and I couldn't have been more grateful for their professionalism, spirit, kindness, and way of treating our son as if he were their own.

So whenever I spotted Dr. Martin anywhere around the hospital and had an opportunity to talk with him face to face, it was a total and complete drop-everything-else code-red priority for me. All other conversations ceased. Sandwiches stopped being eaten. The Blackberry went away. And all incoming phone calls, presidential or otherwise, went directly to voice mail. For the record, if I had known exactly where on Pennsylvania Avenue that particular call originated, hospital VIP or not, I suspect I might have called an audible and amended the Martin Rule just once and taken the call.

Ironically, even with the approaching operation, Dr. Martin and I were not in a deep discussion about the intricacies of the surgery, overnight monitor readings, or how long Paulie needed to stay in the hospital to recover. Nope. We were talking about—of all things—golf. Cardiology honcho or not, like just about every golfer I have ever known, Dr. Martin was regaling me about his love for and frustration with the sport at the exact same time. Apparently the good doctor was

getting off the tee just fine, but his short irons were caus-ing him a bit of a problem.

It was great to have a lighter moment and not be pummeling Dr. Martin with the normal barrage of con-genital heart defect questions I typically hit him with whenever I spotted him anywhere around the hospital, including the restrooms and parking garage.

Knowing how much I love golf, and in a complete re-versal of roles, Dr. Martin was now hitting me up with questions about proper ball position for shorter irons and how to hit a fairway bunker shot without chunking it. In a hopeful glimpse of some future normalcy, he and I were even talking about getting a game together on his home course after Paulie had recovered and was settled in back home.

Apart from lighting up when she heard the words "Paulie," "recovered," "settled," and "home" in the same sentence, it would be safe to say Amy was not into that coffee shop consultation as much as Dr. Martin and I were. Stressed out hospital mom or not—and perhaps with her own attempt at some blessed normalcy—Amy made no pretense about her complete disinterest in the entire conversation.

It was a rare and much needed bit of stress-relieving hallway levity with the man to whom Amy and I were so indebted. But the fact remained: I had just missed a call from the president of the United States, the number-one newsmaker on the planet, commander in chief, and the guy I happened to get paid to cover. I knew White House press secretary Tony Snow or his number two, Dana Perino, probably made that call happen, so I made a mental note to thank them the next time I received an e-mail with their daily request for a Paulie update.

Having never before received a phone call from the president of the United States, I was pretty clueless about the proper protocol for returning said call. I was fairly certain I probably couldn't simply call the White House operators back and say, "Hey, guys. Sorry I missed the president. I was talking to a really important doctor friend of mine about chunking his short irons. I'm sure the president wanted me to call him right back. Can you put me through to the Oval Office?"

To keep it somewhat in perspective, Amy and I had been conversing pretty much hourly with a much higher authority figure over the past twelve days. A conversation with the president—in the grand scheme of things—might not be that big a deal. But Democrat, Republican, or Independent, the president of the United States is still considered the leader of the free world, after all.

On second thought, missing the president's call might have been a complete blessing in disguise. Despite Amy's dialed-in and in-the-zone single-minded devotion to tending to her son, she would certainly be grateful to add another name, presidential or otherwise, to the growing list of people who were praying for Paulie. And as long as my thick fingers could stay away from the delete button on my phone, I had all the physical proof I needed and wouldn't have to spend the rest of the night trying to convince Amy I didn't make the whole thing up.

Apart from having ample forensic evidence in the court of Amy, I was glad to have the president's words on tape for a different reason altogether. I had a vision of one day being able to play that message for Paulie when he was older and he might understand what all the fuss

was about. Perhaps a bit of a fanciful dream, but one day when all this hospital drama had faded into distant memory, maybe I could use the audio on that tape as part of a *This Is Your Life* rehearsal dinner video at Paulie's wedding somewhere around the year 2037.

Maybe Paulie would one day have the opportunity to play the message for his own son or daughter and tell him or her about that time long ago when he had to spend a few days in the hospital for some long-forgotten medical procedure. Nice thoughts, but maybe I was getting a little ahead of myself.

It was not 2037. It was Wednesday, July 11, 2007—just one day before twelve-day-old Paulie would be going into the operating room for open-heart surgery at the hands of Dr. Richard Jonas. Amy and I would be meeting Dr. Jonas for the first time in about ten minutes. And despite our nervousness about the impending operation, we were both feeling somewhat upbeat as we made our way to his office not far from the CICU.

Paulie had successfully made it twelve full days, hanging in there long enough for Dr. Jonas to get back into town. "What spunk and fight this kid has!" I thought. Granted, Paulie was receiving top-notch medical care at a great hospital. And all those prayers and good thoughts flooding in from family, friends—even complete strangers—were really making a difference. But deep down, I had the sense Paulie was doing the heaviest lifting of all. Sometimes it was impossible not to tear up as I looked at him lying there in that hospital bed, knowing the intense life-and-death battle he was waging. I prayed for the day when I would be able to talk to him, father to son, and let him know how proud I was of him and his fighting spirit.

Amy and I were upbeat about reaching day number twelve for a very practical reason, too. Less than fifteen hours before the operation, even if Paulie took an unexpected turn for the worse in the coming overnight hours, Dr. Jonas was at least back in town and could jump into the OR and do the surgery if he had to. Sure, it might still be a scary, middle-of-the-night drama for all concerned, but the operation could be performed at Children's and wouldn't involve a 3:00 a.m. helicopter flight to Philadelphia, Boston, or anywhere else.

Despite all the worst-case scenarios my mind was constantly mulling over, Amy and I had great expectation and hope that with tomorrow's surgery we were going to take a giant leap forward in our goal to finally be able to take Paulie home. Unfortunately, our expectation and hope was constantly being tested and roped back in by the daily reminders that Paulie was still an intensive care patient with a very long way to go.

Although Paulie's little body was growing stronger every day, the amount of oxygen getting to his blood was declining. The doctors warned us this would happen. But still, our hearts jumped every time we heard one of those scary close-to-the-danger-zone alarms coming from his monitor and the nurses had to make a mad dash to his bedside to check things out.

Also, by midweek, the doctors determined Paulie was working his fragile heart way too hard when he sucked milk from the baby bottle. Just a few days before his surgery, they decided it would be much safer to insert a feeding tube into his nose and run it directly to his stomach. Amy and I were a little traumatized by the change in the way Paulie was being fed, not to mention the fact that he had yet another tube going into his lit-

tle body. But in a world where traumas were starting to stack on top of each other like bricks in a LEGOLAND skyscraper, we deferred to the doctors, knowing they were on top of the situation and aware of what Paulie needed.

One more day till surgery—*one more day*.

It was difficult to comprehend everything that had transpired over the past two weeks. Even though we believed Paulie was exactly where he needed to be hospitalwise and was receiving amazing care, the more we thought about the specifics of the operation, the more anxious we got.

The surgery, we were told, would last anywhere from four to eight hours. We were also told Paulie's heart would be completely stopped, and he would be kept alive during the surgery by a heart-lung machine. The idea that Paulie would be kept alive by a machine while a surgeon cut on his walnut-size heart and arteries no bigger than fishing line—well, let's just say it focuses the mind.

As tough as the past two weeks had been on the entire family, if things went our way during the surgery, Amy and I were hopeful that after a week or two recovering in the hospital we might be able to take Paulie home. We counted our blessings knowing that was a very real possibility. Unfortunately, that was not the case for many of the families we met at Children's that week.

Our new friend Maggie and her family had been living this kind of drama not for two weeks like us, or even two months. They had been doing this for nine straight months. They had been on pins and needles for months in the CICU waiting room hoping and praying that Maggie's long string of surgeries would soon end and they would finally be able to take her home.

Whenever I had the opportunity to talk with Maggie's parents, I was always impressed by their forbearance, stamina, and pure love for their little girl. I knew what Amy and I were feeling about Paulie's upcoming surgery—hopefully his last. I couldn't imagine what Maggie's parents had been going through over the past nine months. Watching them day after day in the CICU and around the hospital, I truly believed the only way they could possibly be getting through this ordeal was by the grace of God. I decided that if God's grace and sustenance had carried Maggie's parents through nine surgeries in nine months, surely the Lord must have enough of a supply to take care of the Baier family for one more day.

We knew the overriding question about Paulie's surgery was whether Dr. Jonas would be able to perform a complete, one-time fix, or whether Paulie would need additional surgeries down the road. The unknown had to do with whether there was enough room in Paulie's chest cavity to do a "patch" using his own arteries, or whether Dr. Jonas would have to sew in a connector called a homograph—essentially, a temporary work-around that would need to be replaced within a few years.

The connector—a donated aorta from another newborn—would eventually need to be replaced because it wouldn't be able to grow along with the rest of Paulie's body. In fact, if Dr. Jonas had to go the route of using a donated aorta, we were probably looking at three to four additional open-heart surgeries throughout Paulie's childhood. We, of course, were hoping and praying for the one-time fix, but we really had no idea how realistic that scenario was.

Despite the anxiety Amy and I felt as the final hours clicked down, we were both pretty excited about finally being able to meet Dr. Jonas in person. By now we were convinced that not only was he the man who was going to save our son's life, he was going to give Paulie a decent shot at a future. Back in town after being away for two weeks, Dr. Jonas was backed up with surgeries from the minute he walked in the door. Wednesday, one day before the surgery, was the first real opportunity we had to sit down with him and discuss specifics about Paulie's heart.

We were told Dr. Jonas had been fully briefed on Paulie's case while he was overseas via e-mail communication with members of Children's cardiology team. Knowing the extreme complexities of Paulie's heart, Dr. Jonas wanted a few extra days after he got back so he could consult with the echocardiographers and determine the best way to approach the surgery before he sat down and talked to us about specifics.

Getting on Dr. Jonas's schedule, for babies or parents, is a bit of a tricky proposition. Because he is one of the best pediatric heart surgeons in the world, parents from all over the globe bring their babies and young children to him year-round so he can work his miracles on their deformed or wrongly wired hearts. Families from the Middle East, Europe, Asia, and of course all over the United States regularly travel to Children's National Medical Center specifically because it is where Dr. Jonas and his team are based.

Performing approximately 350 highly complex heart surgeries each year, Dr. Jonas often does two, sometimes three surgeries a day, including heart transplants. With international travel schedules, family accommodations

required, and the intricacies of transporting sick babies with very fragile hearts, many of those surgeries need to be scheduled months in advance so the myriad of logistical details can be worked out.

However, despite his always-packed surgery calendar, Children's, thankfully, builds in open spaces on Dr. Jonas's schedule so newborns like Paulie can undergo emergency procedures without totally disrupting the plans of all those other families who are continually cycling in for their children's long-scheduled operations.

Given his hectic, nonstop schedule, Amy and I didn't expect to have more than a few minutes with Dr. Jonas. As he had already performed two surgeries that day, one in the morning and one in the afternoon, our meeting was scheduled to take place in his office after he was done operating for the day.

Since Paulie had five separate complex congenital issues, Dr. Jonas needed to meet with us to go over the details of not only how he was going to approach the overall operation but also how he planned to sequence the various procedures he needed to perform. We had been forewarned that he also needed to talk to us about the risks associated with performing surgery on such a small structure as Paulie's heart, not to mention the complexities created by a heart with multiple abnormalities.

Because of his stellar reputation, all the stories we had heard, and the long buildup to finally meeting him, Amy and I half expected to find ourselves walking down a long, ornate *Wizard of Oz* hallway leading to a massive space-age–looking office with a floor-to-ceiling video wall, three-dimensional holographic heart models floating in the air, and a clear glass tube transporter reserved

for superhero surgeons who need to appear in the OR at a moment's notice.

In reality, once we arrived at Dr. Jonas's fairly normal-looking and normal-size office, we were escorted to a nondescript conference room nearby with a table, eight chairs, and a white erasable board with green drawings on it. No high-tech monitors. No holographic heart models. No funky high-speed transporter. Just two very nervous parents sitting at a conference table looking at a white erasable board with green drawings that made no sense at all.

Entering the room, Dr. Jonas smiled and asked, "How are you both holding up?"

Dr. Jonas was tan, fit, and had a distinguished head of silvery gray hair and a hybrid Australian/Boston accent, with maybe a little something else thrown in just to confuse people. More Australian than Bostonian, I decided, but he definitely had a northeast cadence when he spoke, I thought. Soft-spoken and calm, Dr. Jonas didn't seem rushed in the least. His demeanor was disarmingly engaging and pleasant.

Having been with him for less than ninety seconds, I started to understand how this Miracle Surgeon who performed some of the world's most complicated surgeries wound up on everyone's Best lists. Dr. Jonas exudes an easy, informal, approachable confidence with zero drama. In talking with him, I quickly got the impression he had Paulie's heart figured out and couldn't wait to get in there to see it and fix it. Although he didn't say these exact words, everything about his demeanor and spirit calmly and quietly whispered, "No worries, mate."

With two complicated, lifesaving surgeries already checked off on his to-do list that day, if someone had

poked their head into the conference room to tell him he had to do two more, including a transplant, I got the idea Dr. Jonas would have smiled and said, "No problem. Be right there." Dr. Jonas has a unique calming quality that is extraordinary, given not only his line of work but also the fact that he must often sit across conference tables from totally stressed-out parents worried sick about their children. Within two or three minutes, Amy and I were completely at ease, and a huge load had been lifted from our shoulders.

We obviously knew open-heart surgery on a baby is not a walk in the park for the baby or the surgeon, superhero or not. The more Dr. Jonas spoke, I got the sense that, as complex as Paulie's case was, everything was under control and he would get the job done despite any challenges that might present themselves once he started operating.

Drawing a picture of Paulie's heart on a piece of paper, Dr. Jonas explained that he had met with the rest of the cardiac team and had mapped out the broad strokes of how he was going to proceed. He said he wouldn't have the complete picture until he actually got in there and saw for himself. The night before he performs surgery, Dr. Jonas said he typically spends the evening drawing out exactly what he is going to do the next day, then runs that scenario over and over in his mind as if he were watching a movie. His mind continues rehearsing the operation all night long while he is literally sleeping on it, he said.

Getting to the key question of the one-time fix, Dr. Jonas told us he would not have an answer until he got in there and saw how much room there was in Paulie's chest cavity. Even though the pictures from the echocar-

diogram team were 100 percent accurate, Dr. Jonas said they were still only two-dimensional, and the one-time-fix comes down to a matter of millimeters one way or the other.

Perfect in his presentation and demeanor, Dr. Jonas exuded hope and confidence. Unfortunately, as we expected, he soon segued into the obligatory talk about legalities and percentages regarding what could go wrong during the operation. I just as quickly segued into a dual case of lump in throat and pit in stomach disease. I could see Amy was similarly afflicted.

Dr. Jonas explained that, though rare, there was a chance Paulie's heart would not start again once he came off the heart-lung machine. He said there was also a chance Paulie could develop excessive bleeding during the surgery or possibly pick up an infection, both of which could prove to be fatal.

Each one of the fatality scenarios Dr. Jonas mentioned had a specific percentage attached to it. And while most of the percentages didn't rise above a 1 or 2 percent risk factor, to my mind there seemed to be about five hundred separate things that could possibly go wrong. My English and Political Science major's mind was working overtime trying to keep up with all the math. But being somewhat of a big-picture guy and someone who is always looking to simplify and sum up, I finally settled on the idea that even with all the risk factors associated with such a complicated operation, without surgery Paulie had zero chance for survival. Focusing on that part of the equation trumped most of the fears I had about any of the what-could-go-wrong percentages.

After finishing the obligatory risks and percentages part of the consultation, Dr. Jonas, still with his calm

Australian demeanor, smiled and softly said, "Look. I don't believe any of those things are going to happen. Make no mistake about it, this is a very complex case, and I can't tell you exactly how I am going to do everything until I get in there. But if all goes the way I think it will, Paulie will be on the road to recovery tomorrow afternoon with a fixed and working heart."

That's all I needed to hear. I immediately signed the consent forms, stood up, and shook Dr. Jonas's hand— *very softly*. In tears, Amy gave Dr. Jonas a big hug. I thought, "Honey, don't squeeze him too hard. And please watch out for those hands!" It was a very emotional moment for both of us. Seriously, if Paulie got through this surgery and Dr. Jonas was successful in putting him on the road to recovery, I would come back and give him a big Baier hug of my own.

Immediately after we met with Dr. Jonas, Amy and I walked back to the CICU to check on Paulie. Before long, I slipped out to my communications command post in the waiting room so I could update all our prayer warriors about the big day tomorrow and make sure everyone knew we needed them suited up and on the field by 7:30 a.m.

July 11, 2007, 6:34 PM, Wednesday
Subject: A patient little patient

Thank you all for your continued e-mails of encouragement, your thoughts, and your prayers. We're finally about to embark on the scariest part of this journey so far—the surgery itself and then the recovery. Our little Paul (who is now 12 days old) is scheduled to go into surgery early Thursday morning.

Right now, the surgeons believe they will be able to try what is called a complete repair, which would mean only one surgery. Obviously, there are a number of things that could change once the surgery begins, but one surgery fixing the defects and blockages in and around his heart is what we have been hoping and praying for so we can start our little guy on the road to recovery.

Paul's been a little fighter from the beginning, and it has been a real blessing to be able to hold him and show him love in these days ahead of surgery. While he's managed to grow and to get stronger, Amy had to stop breast-feeding him and then had to stop feeding him by the bottle since it was producing too much stress for his heart, which happens to be working extra hard to pump blood to and from the lungs in the WRONG way. It's amazing that his body taught itself to adapt to his defects that quickly. So Paul has been on a feeding tube for the past few days. He's still getting Mom's breast milk, but it's being fed into his stomach every four hours.

We've spent 12 to 15-hour days at Children's National Medical Center in D.C. in the Cardiac Intensive Care Unit. The doctors and nurses are top notch, extremely impressive and extremely caring. Every patient is "one of their children." We could not be in better hands. When we are not at the hospital, we have backup. What we have come to call the Grandma Brigade has reported for duty. We call Grandma Baier and Grandma Hills a brigade because that sounds more official. They have been holding Paul, singing to him, telling him stories, and showering him with affection. We've also had uncles and aunts streaming in as well. Every day ends with me turning to Amy and giving her a

high five, saying, "We're one day closer to getting Paulie home!"

This is the final update e-mail I will send prior to surgery. I don't mean to bombard you with e-mails, but a number of you have asked for more updates, so I thought I would send another. This one comes with one more request to please keep Paul in your thoughts and prayers—especially early Thursday morning. Depending on how everything goes, the surgery could take anywhere from four to eight hours. We're told the next 48 to 72 hours after surgery are critical and will determine how his body is reacting to the procedure. Hopefully, by next week we'll have some good news to share.

Paul is the best thing that has ever happened to us. And we can't wait to get him home!

Thank you again for your support.

Bret and Amy

Not much sleep during the night. Amy and I awoke at about 5:00 a.m. and decided to head into the hospital early. Dr. Jonas told us the anesthesiology team would come around 7:30 a.m., and his part would begin about an hour later, after Paulie was fully anesthetized and properly positioned on the operating table. The rest of the Baier–Hills family was going to be at Children's during the surgery, and later in the morning Father Kevin O'Brien from our local parish was go-

ing to come in and hold a prayer service for us in the hospital chapel.

Arriving at Paulie's bedside in the CICU around 6:30 a.m., before long the anesthesiologist, Dr. Songyos Valairucha—Dr. V, as everyone called him—came in and introduced himself. An extremely affable guy, I'm sure Dr. V could see we were stressed beyond belief. He, like Dr. Jonas, had a very calm demeanor and was very pleasant and reassuring. Dr. V explained exactly what was going to happen to Paulie to get him ready for the surgery.

Like Dr. Jonas, Dr. Valairucha had his own list of things that could go wrong: might slip into a coma and not wake up, could stop breathing during surgery and die, could suffer lasting brain damage, could have negative reaction to anesthesia, or any number of other fine-print complications.

As with Dr. Jonas, after we had been given all the information about the risks associated with putting Paulie under for such a long and complicated surgery, we had to sign another round of consent forms. Lots of scary scenarios raced through my mind. Thankfully, I was constantly returning to my self-styled mantra: the biggest risk for Paulie is to not take a risk and deny him the chance to get beyond all this.

As they prepared to take Paulie away, I could see that Amy was tensing up. I turned to her and said, "Time to turn him over now—to the doctors and to the big Guy upstairs." Amy nodded. Dr. V said he would take good care of Paulie. And he repeated what everyone had been telling us all week: "Paulie will be in good hands. Dr. Jonas is great!"

We kissed Paulie good-bye. Whispering in his little ear one final time, Amy said, "We'll see you in a few

hours, peanut." I held Paulie's little fingers in mine, and Amy kissed him one more time on the forehead. Then the doctors and nurses assisting Dr. Jonas rolled Paulie's medical bassinet away and down the hall toward the hospital's Joe Robert Surgical Center.

A tough moment. Amy and I hugged each other, wiped away a few tears, and then decided to walk to what we now considered to be our own little chapel to pray, not far from the CICU waiting room. Amy and I had spent a lot of time in that chapel over the past twelve days, always seeming to find it empty whenever we needed it most.

Before we left the CICU, one of the nurses handed me a pager that she said we should keep with us throughout the surgery. She told us we would receive pages at various stages of Paulie's operation so we could have a sense of where Dr. Jonas was in the procedure in real time. She said we would receive a page when Paulie's chest was opened, when he was put on the heart-lung machine, when he came off the heart-lung machine, and finally when the surgery was completed.

Under any other circumstance I am sure I would have been extremely interested in all the gizmos they were using and pages they were planning to send. But being more Dad than reporter at that point, I wasn't sure I wanted to know that much detail in real time. Moments in time that I interpreted less delicately as when they cut open his chest, when his heart stops beating, when his body is being run by a machine, when his heart starts beating again, and when they stitch him up. After my initial hesitation about taking the pager, I soon found myself looking down and checking it every thirty seconds to make sure it was working properly.

Amy and I held hands as we made our way to the chapel. Trying to maintain some level of calm, I avoided looking at the clocks on the waiting room wall, knowing any second hand we saw would be marching toward the moment when Dr. Jonas would start cutting open Paulie's chest. Soon we met up with the rest of the family and Father Kevin for a small service in the chapel. Nothing fancy, but we prayed for Dr. Jonas and his team, for Paulie, and for strength for the entire family. Father Kevin read a few verses from the Bible then gave us a blessing. Based on the e-mails I was receiving, Amy and I took great comfort knowing so many people were praying for Paulie that morning and would continue throughout the entire operation.

After the chapel service we camped out in the waiting room area with an occasional trip to the cafeteria to get coffee, all the while looking at that hospital pager:

—Chest opened
—Now on heart-lung machine
—Off heart-lung machine

Minutes turned to hours, and eventually the hospital pager buzzed one final time:

—Surgery completed—please meet Dr. Jonas in waiting room.

July 12, 2007, 11:49 PM, Thursday
Subject: The longest day

After almost six hours of heart surgery today, our thirteen-day-old son Paul is recovering tonight and doing better than

anyone expected him to be doing. Thank you all for your thoughts and prayers—we think they helped a great deal today.

Paul started his surgery at 8:30 a.m. He then went on a heart-lung machine, which bypassed his own body's control about an hour and a half later. Shortly after 1:30 p.m., he came off the bypass and was finished with surgery at almost 2:30 p.m.

This was the longest, most stressful day of our lives.

Dr. Richard Jonas, Paul's surgeon—a world-renowned specialist in the field—came out of surgery and took Amy and me to a small conference room outside of the Operating Room. I could hear my heart beating loudly in my eardrums. Amy held her chest—trying to get her heart to stop beating as fast as it was. We didn't say a word. We knew it would be hard to focus on every detail. But, we had been preparing all day for Dr. Jonas's first few words to us.

As Dr. Jonas closed the door of the small conference room, we both held our breath. Time stood still. It was a slow-motion movie as we watched him close the door and sit down at the table in front of us. I will always remember his first two sentences:

"I believe the surgery went exceptionally well"—a first sentence that triggered a giant exhale from both of us. But that glorious sentence was followed by an ominous one. "This was as long and as complicated as any surgery we've done."

This from a surgeon who performs more than 350 heart surgeries a year and whose team is shuttled around the world to fix hearts on every continent.

And the next sentence was equally tough to hear. Dr. Jonas said, "We couldn't do the one-time fix. There simply wasn't enough room in there. But Paul did very well."

So that means, beyond this fix, there will be more hurdles ahead, but the first real hurdle is the next 48 hours—that's our real focus now. Paul is far from out of the woods tonight. The next two days will be critical to see how Paul's body deals with the changes Dr. Jonas made to his heart.

Paul's chest is still open tonight, and it's covered with a clear bandage through which you can actually SEE his heart beating. And that tiny walnut-size heart is beating. I must have stared at it for at least 30 minutes straight—fascinated and frightened but encouraged, thanking God that it's still beating and for the medical miracle that has enabled Paul to be alive, yet deathly afraid that at any second that heart could stop beating. It's mesmerizing, awe-inspiring, and terrifying all in one.

There are a host of things that COULD happen, but right now our little guy is fighting hard and doing extremely well. Late tonight, Dr. Jonas stopped by the Cardiac Intensive Care Unit to check on Paul, almost seven hours after surgery. Right now, Paul's heart is beating on its own without the use of heavy drugs or other means. ALL of his vital signs look good tonight. The same man who uttered those first two crucial sentences postsurgery—one that triggered an exhale, and

another that triggered a gulp—gave us two more sen-tences tonight that triggered a determined smile:

"Paul is doing better right now than ninety-nine percent of our patients following surgery—let alone a surgery of that length. He's really looking strong now."

Dr. Jonas grew up in Australia but has lived in Boston for a long time so he has an interesting Australian/Bostonian ac-cent that to me comes off as very calming and reassuring, yet he is always straightforward and to the point. Tonight, we got the point: Paul is doing very well! We have a long road ahead, but the first hurdle is behind us. And it was a big one. The fact that a surgeon can operate for seven hours on a walnut-size heart and fix at least five major problems, then put that heart on the road to recovery, bog-gles my mind. It also bolsters my faith in modern medicine and in God.

After Paul went to surgery this morning, Father Kevin O'Brien from our parish, Holy Trinity in Georgetown, came to the hospital and led a prayer service in the hospital's chapel for my family. It meant a great deal to us and really helped us get through what was an extremely tough day.

I want to thank everyone who has been pulling for us, think-ing of us and praying for us. It's meant the world to our family. Paul is a fighter, and we're gonna make it, one step at a time. We're far from being in the clear, and we will likely have a rocky road ahead, but we feel blessed to be where we are and to have great friends and family standing be-hind us and supporting us.

And tonight when we left the hospital I turned to Amy and gave her a teary-eyed high five, saying: "We are one day closer to bringing Paulie home!" And this was the longest one yet.

I will share one other thing. As we have obviously been focused on Paulie, there are many other families in our situation or worse at Children's National Medical Center. We have been fortunate enough to meet and talk with some of them. The strength and resilience of these families has been an inspiration to us. Many of their children have more than heart problems—they have liver, kidney, stomach, or other problems as well.

We met one family whose nine-month-old daughter, Maggie, had been through nine surgeries in those nine months. The family has been at Children's pretty much nonstop since April. We spent a lot of time over the past twelve days "in the trenches" of the waiting room with them. We walked by Maggie's bedside every day on the way to see Paul and we talked frequently with her family about Maggie's many health issues and how they had fought them off one by one.

Well, Maggie ended her battle last night—she died after her kidneys failed.

We found out this morning when we arrived to an empty waiting room—a room that had been filled with anxious family members—pulling for Maggie and helping each other—staying overnight every night to be at her bedside. It was devastating news. We have been here only twelve days, but we now feel a part of the "Children's family." And that family has taken a big hit with Maggie's death.

Tonight after Paul's surgery as we were standing next to his bassinet looking at his heart beat through his chest, a CICU nurse told me I had a phone call. I took it at a phone a few feet from Paul's bed. It was Maggie's mom. She wanted to check on Paul—to see how he did in surgery. I gave her an update and then passed on our condolences to her family. I told her we know Maggie is in a very peaceful place now. I told her that her family was a true inspiration to us as we begin this tough journey. A mother who had just lost her daughter hours before called us to check on our son after his heart surgery. The power, the grace, and the strength it took to make that call! We are truly humbled.

The past twelve days have given us an amazing new perspective on life. Thank you all for being there for us. And may God bless Maggie's family tonight.

Sincerely,
Bret and Amy

CHAPTER EIGHT

Miracles Do Happen

It was just before 1:00 a.m. Friday, July 20, and I was about to jump out of my skin. Amy and I had been back from the hospital for more than two hours, but I was so excited about bringing Paulie home tomorrow—*later today*—I couldn't even think about going to bed yet. Three weeks after he was diagnosed with life-threatening congenital heart defects, and just eight days after undergoing what Dr. Richard Jonas called one of the most complicated surgeries he has ever performed, we were finally going to bring Paulie home from the hospital.

Although we didn't get the "one-time fix" we were hoping and praying for, all the doctors were greatly encouraged about the results of Paulie's surgery, and especially his rapid recovery. Not only was he ahead of schedule in hitting all the important postsurgery milestones required before he could be discharged, but the doctors said he was recovering faster than just about any baby they had ever seen following such a long and complicated heart operation. In fact, Paulie was out of the

Cardiac Intensive Care Unit just four days after surgery and was now in a private room one floor above the CICU.

Even though we knew he would need future open-heart surgeries and his world would be one of constant poking, prodding, catheterizations, angioplasties, hospital stays, checkups, blood samples, treadmill tests, and continual monitoring, Amy and I were humbled and thankful to God that Paulie's life had been spared and that he had at least a shot at living a normal little boy's life.

The cardiologists at Children's had already told us Paulie would need at least one catheterization or angioplasty in five or six months, followed by a second open-heart surgery sometime after that. But Amy and I were trying not to think about future operations or hospital stays just yet. Paulie had just fought his way through an incredibly complex, six-hour open-heart surgery with flying colors. Given the Baier family's stress-o-rama of the past three weeks, Amy and I desperately needed a little time and space to celebrate getting through this first operation before we faced the reality of future ones.

Once we got Paulie home, Amy and I pledged to do our best not to obsess about the unknowns and instead enjoy the known-known we had right here, right now. And what we had—or *would* have in about thirteen hours and twenty-seven minutes, depending on whether I got lost driving—was our son, Paul Francis Baier, home at last. That was all Amy and I wanted right now—nothing more.

Even with all the question marks about Paulie's future surgeries and hospital stays, the prospect of four or five months of nonhospital, uneventful normalcy seemed

pretty wonderful to us. We were eagerly looking forward to picking up where we left off three weeks ago when the Three Baiers' bonding process was interrupted at Sibley Hospital after we learned that our adorable and perfect baby boy didn't have such a perfect heart.

For me, the thought of now being able to snuggle with Paulie in our own home and on our own couch without tubes, wires, and the omnipresent beeps and buzzes of the CICU seemed like heaven come down to earth.

While I was wide awake and bouncing off the walls of the condo with excited anticipation about the upcoming day, Amy, thankfully, had drifted off and was catching some sleep. Physically and emotionally drained, she had to get up in just a few hours for her middle-of-the-night breast pumping. I was amazed at how disciplined she had been in keeping up with that, especially given the nonstop emotional roller-coaster ride of the past three weeks. Whether she was here at the condo or over at Children's, every four hours Amy was pumping and freezing milk for Paulie.

Typically, after we returned home from the hospital around 11:00 p.m. every night, Amy would sit in the rocker next to Paulie's crib and pump before she went to bed. After a few hours' sleep, she would be at it again around three in the morning. Hoping to squeeze in a few hours of sleep before the sun came up, Amy would wake up around 7:00 a.m. and pump once more before we headed out the door to Children's for the day.

Amy's tenacity and faithfulness were really paying dividends. Even with his complicated heart and blood oxygen issues, by all indicators Paulie was growing like a weed. There was a huge upside for Amy, too. Despite the craziness and uncertainty of the past twenty-one

days, those appointments every four hours turned out to be a welcome constant in her life, a comforting ritual that helped Amy maintain some semblance of normalcy—even serenity—in the midst of the storm.

Because she was also pumping throughout the day at Children's, there was never really any need for us to tap into our home freezer supply and take milk pouches into the hospital. After three straight weeks of Amy's round-the-clock devotion to her motherly duties we had accumulated quite a supply. Our small freezer was packed to the roof with plastic milk pouches marked with the dates and times Amy had clocked in over the past three weeks. I had no idea how long breast milk would keep, but if Amy kept at this much longer we were going to have to buy a bigger freezer, open a dairy farm, or get some kind of auction going on eBay.

During some of the toughest moments over the past three weeks, while Amy was breast pumping in Paulie's room, I would hear her trying to hold back the sad tears of a mother pining for her child. That was all about to change. Just hours before Paulie would finally be home with us, I knew Amy's upcoming shift in the rocker would be accompanied by a big smile.

We were both doing a lot of smiling lately.

Standing next to Paulie's crib, I grinned as I imagined being in this identical spot tomorrow night at about this same time, holding a screaming baby and loving every blessed minute of it. No amount of kicking and screaming in the middle of the night could ever be as nerve-racking and deafening as the sounds of Paulie not being there with us over the past weeks. And with the record-setting decibel levels he seemed to be achieving lately at Children's, we definitely were going to be

able to give our neighbor Rob Jewell's sound system a run for its money in the late-night music department. I wondered how long it would take for me—not to mention Rob—to stop loving every blessed minute of it.

Trying to be as quiet as possible and not wake Amy, in a time-honored ritual known to all first-time parents, I nervously flitted around the condo babyproofing the place for probably the billionth time. You can't be too careful about these things. You never know; three-week-old Paulie just might climb out of his crib, crawl into the living room, leap seven feet up to the chandelier, and start practicing his baby trapeze stunts. Better get the ladder out and check those ceiling bolts one more time to be safe.

I knew the plastic set of golf clubs I put in the corner of the crib might not pass muster with the U.S. Consumer Product Safety Commission. But Paulie had just survived a hypercomplicated six-hour surgery that basically rebuilt his heart from scratch, not to mention three weeks in intensive care. In the grand scheme of things I didn't think a three-ounce miniature plastic putter falling over on him presented too much of a challenge.

Being in the room where we would soon be spending serious bonding time with our son, I decided to get Amy's rocker warm and ready for her upcoming shift. One o'clock in the morning or not, I was so overflowing with gratitude and joy that this day had finally come that I couldn't keep my excitement bottled up any longer. I grabbed my laptop and wrote a message of thanks to our family, friends, and colleagues who had been standing with us over the past weeks and gave them an update on the miracle child who by now was inspiring us all.

July 20, 2007, 1:00 AM, Friday
Subject: Miracles DO happen!

Thank you all for your concern—the e-mails, letters, well wishes, thoughts, and most of all the prayers have been fantastic, and needless to say much APPRECIATED! I am sorry I haven't written to update everyone on Paul's recovery. Honestly, I have been trying not to jinx it or screw it up in some way by sending out an update before we are home with him.

I have knocked on every piece of wood I pass by. But it's time to share the good news. Paul's doctors and nurses at Children's National Medical Center have told us that Paulie is coming home Friday afternoon! One week and one day after what his surgeon called the "longest and most complex" heart surgery his team has done, Paul's heart is working well—actually, it's working extremely well.

The doctors have been shaking their heads in disbelief about the speed and success of Paulie's recovery. I feel nervous that I just typed that, but multiple doctors and nurses have told us the same thing. (I am knocking on this desk now. I know—it's stupid.) But—come on! Just eight days after I stared, fascinated and terrified at the same time, into my son's open chest through a clear bandage to watch his beating heart, he is coming home! Just him. No equipment, just seven-pound him and the best-looking chest scar we have ever seen.

Immediately after the surgery, we were told about all of these hurdles that Paulie would need to get over to get to the "next stage" of recovery (e.g., he needed to urinate a

lot, or he needed to breathe on his own for a certain amount of time, or he needed to start eating out of a bottle). Paul passed all of those tests with flying colors DAYS, if not weeks, ahead of schedule. He was out of intensive care in a record four days after surgery.

The people who work at Children's are extremely caring and very good at what they do. All of them obviously try not to cause pain to the child. But part of the recovery process involves constant prodding, poking, sticking, blood testing, weighing, attaching wires, adding tubes, detaching other wires to add other wires, changing more tubes, and applying sticky tape to hold it all on Paul's tiny little frame. Paulie's a fair-skinned part-Irishman who doesn't take to the tape too well.

All of the things they are doing are essential to make sure his heart is doing what it's supposed to be doing. Well, Paul had had enough of it by about day three postsurgery, and he let his doctors and nurses know it every single time. Paul got a lot of lung practice during the past week. He's definitely going to win the "I can swim to the other side of the pool underwater contest" when he's a little older.

The funny part is, after the doctors or nurses are finished and he's screamed so loud the next floor takes notice, Paul then chills out completely like nothing has happened. He sucks on his pacifier and saves his strength for the next bout with another wire-fixer or tube-tweaker. To put it simply, he has heart.

We can't thank Dr. Richard Jonas and his staff enough for the work they did on Paul's walnut-size heart. I won't go into too

much detail here, but there were five major congenital defects in Paul's heart, an extremely rare combination. Added to that, one of the main fixes was not possible because of the way Paul's coronary arteries crisscrossed his heart.

So part of the six-hour surgery involved attaching a donor baby aorta to Paul's heart (specifically his right ventricle), then linking that donor aorta to his pulmonary artery, essentially rerouting the blood over the top of the crisscrossed arteries like a major highway overpass. The conduit was a tiny tube from another baby who died and whose parents agreed to allow that baby to be an organ donor so our baby could live.

It's an amazing thought: a selfless decision made by one family during a moment of ultimate grief provides another unknown family ultimate joy after their darkest hours. In a few years Paul will have at least one more surgery to change that conduit as he grows. But the surgery—or surgeries (he could be a big boy and might require a third surgery as a teen)—will be nowhere near as complicated as the one that he just went through.

I know these e-mails are long, but just a couple more thoughts. I am amazed at how much Paul has managed to DO in his first 21 days of life. He has brought our extended family much closer (they rallied around us from the beginning). He made me love my wife Amy even more than I could have imagined. He opened our eyes to the goodness and caring in so many people, some we barely know, and we've been humbled by their actions and words. He reminded us how fragile life really is. He's inspired us to be better (if he can fight so can we). He showed us just how far

modern medicine has come. And most of all, he renewed our faith and belief in the power of prayer.

We could not have made it through this without our faith, and without the comfort we received knowing that hundreds of people were praying (and are praying) for Paul's recovery. We literally thank God for every single day we have with our son. And I know from dozens of e-mails, Paulie's battle made many fathers and mothers hug their kids a little tighter. Paul has given us all PERSPECTIVE...

Thank you all. This is my last update—I plan to spend any extra time I have getting to know this little guy and enjoying every minute. Amy and I will surely have an anxious road of parenting ahead (especially at the beginning), but all of the teary high fives at the end of the day leaving the hospital and the mantra of "We're one day closer to getting Paulie home" paid off. Today is our day!

Sincerely,
Bret and Amy

With Amy and Paulie nestled in back at the condo and me back at work, the Baier clan could not have been happier or more content. Everyone was exactly where they were supposed to be and doing exactly what they were supposed to be doing. Apart from the fact that the plastic golf clubs kept falling over on Paulie and had to come out of the crib, life could not have been any better for us.

Amy was ecstatic about being a new mom and enjoy-

ing time with her son at home. And Paulie was coming along exceptionally well other than a little difficulty he was having keeping his food down. We got to the point where we had to keep him upright when we were feeding him, otherwise Paulie would often rocket his food back in our direction like he was waiting at the net ready to pounce on a lazy overhand volley. I believe the medical term for this is "projectile vomiting." And although it is not yet an officially sanctioned Olympic event, Paulie definitely seemed interested in going for some kind of distance record. Movie buffs might appreciate knowing that our condo was just a few short blocks from the stairs featured in the 1970s film *The Exorcist*, a fact that entered my head only about every seventeen seconds during Paulie's projectile phase.

Doing her best to stay out of the line of fire, Amy was keeping a close watch on the situation and had spoken to the doctors about it. They said they would look at Paulie the next time Amy brought him in for one of his checkups at Children's. After everything Paulie had been through over the past month, having trouble keeping his food down didn't seem like that big a deal to me, so I didn't worry too much about it as I got back into the groove covering the White House.

My bosses at Fox had been incredibly supportive in giving me all the time off I needed during Paulie's hospitalization. But reporting assignments bureauwide had to be shifted around to cover for me while I was gone, so I was extremely grateful to my colleagues whose schedules and lives were affected by Paulie's hospitalization and my time away from the bureau.

My first day back at the White House, spokesman Tony Snow and all my competitor/colleagues made me

feel right at home when they spotted me in the media work area or the briefing room for the first time. To a person, colleagues from the other networks and newspapers seemed to know something about Paulie's situation. All day long folks were coming up to me wanting to hear the latest. Interestingly, most of the male reporters were extremely interested in the medical details, while the women mostly wanted to know how Paulie and Amy were doing.

Paulie even achieved a bit of nationwide notoriety among the C-SPAN viewing audience when Tony entered the briefing room and spotted me in my normal seat for his 1:00 p.m. televised news conference. The entire exchange made it into the official White House transcript that day.

> **MR. SNOW:** As Bill Plante just said, let's begin by welcoming back Bret Baier. You've been in a lot of our thoughts and prayers, and very happy to hear that Bret's son has come through some very testing surgery, coming through with flying colors. (Applause.) There's no fear like a parent worrying about a kid. So, God bless you. Just very happy to hear it.
> We are going to give you some audio-visuals—or some visuals today.
> **Q:** Oh, boy.
> **Q:** Pictures of Bret's baby? (Laughter.)
> **MR. SNOW:** No, but I'll tell you what, we expect to see those soon.

After the important news of the day about Paulie, Tony took questions on an array of non-Paulie topics

including the ongoing war in Iraq, the military surge, al Qaeda, Pakistan, the Middle East, American citizens being held in Iran, commutation for some imprisoned border patrol agents, nuclear plant security, and the story I was working on my first day back, trade with China.

President Bush had set up something called the Import Safety Working Group, a task force designed to come up with recommendations to minimize dangers from food and other products shipped into the United States. To be perfectly honest, knowing Paulie was recovering and safe at home with Amy, it was nice to be able to transport my mind thousands of miles away from intensive care units and open-heart surgeries for a brief spell, even if it took contaminated Chinese cat food to do it.

The White House was an amazing place to go to work every day. The range of stories was always vast and wide, and power politics between Capitol Hill and the White House was something I had been fascinated by my entire life. It was an honor and privilege to cover the White House for Fox News, and I pinched myself every day just to make sure that was really me sitting there in that briefing room asking questions and covering the stories I was covering.

Truth be told, it was a little ironic I ever wound up working as a reporter at the White House, or anywhere else for that matter.

After I was elected student council president at the Marist School in Atlanta back in the late 1980s, I was chosen to travel to Washington, D.C., with our headmaster, Fr. Joel Konzen, and another teacher to accept a national excellence in education award being given to Marist and several other private schools from across the country.

It was a huge honor for Marist and me to be able to go to Washington, meet President Ronald Reagan, and participate in a ceremony in the White House Rose Garden—a real dream come true. Embossed White House invitation. Rose Garden ceremony. Meeting President Reagan. Seeing the White House press corps up close. All on the same day. Wow! Pretty heady stuff for an idealistic seventeen-year-old high school kid from Georgia.

During the ceremony the president delivered remarks on education and then presented the awards. After pictures were taken and when the event was wrapping up, President Reagan turned and started walking toward the familiar white marble colonnade and back to the Oval Office. Just as the president was leaving, with all the award winners still assembled and basking in the glow of the event, ABC News White House correspondent Sam Donaldson shouted out a question, asking President Reagan if he was going to withdraw his nomination of Judge Robert Bork to the United States Supreme Court.

"Over my dead body," President Reagan replied as he continued walking away.

The reporters continued yelling questions at the president until he disappeared through the door and into the White House. It wasn't long before a few of the school principals started exchanging words with the reporters, accusing them of stepping all over our sacred event. Standing their ground, the reporters charged right back and told the principals the event was over and this was the only chance they had to put their questions to the president.

First Amendment rights trampled on or not, to my

impressionable seventeen-year-old mind, my once-in-a-lifetime moment at the White House was trampled on by Donaldson and the other reporters gathered in the Rose Garden that morning. I was so angry that when I got back to Atlanta I penned an op-ed piece for the Marist school newspaper, *The Blue & Gold*, where I served as sports editor. Titled "Press Needs Etiquette," my editorial took Donaldson and the other reporters to task for their "obnoxious" and "disrespectful" behavior during this solemn ceremony honoring excellence in education, Marist, and, of course, me.

Years later, as I started my second week as Fox News Channel's chief White House correspondent, a former Marist classmate of mine was kind enough to send me a copy of the editorial I wrote all those years ago. On a campaign trip I once met the legendary Donaldson and regaled him with the story and the highlights of my stinging editorial rant. Sam and I had quite a good laugh about that. With raised eyebrow, he quickly asked me, "So how many questions have you had to yell?"

I have to admit I have employed the Donaldson Rule a few times over my career, without yielding the same kind of result Sam got that day in the Rose Garden in 1987. Shouted questions seldom yield much news, but occasionally every White House reporter has to do it, especially if a president isn't holding regular news conferences or is being evasive on a particular issue.

I obviously have a different take on things now than I did as an idealistic student council president trying to soak in all the pomp and circumstance of a White House Rose Garden ceremony. Now, with the instant and never-ending constancy of the Internet, most White House reporters are editorialized and beat up on

regularly—sometimes hourly—for the questions they ask, don't ask, should have asked, forgot to ask, were too afraid to ask, and on and on. My only advice to any aspiring young journalist who might aim to one day be a news reporter in Washington? Think twice before writing those editorials. They surely will come back to haunt you!

For the record, with the long lead times required for school newspapers and before the Internet came along, by the time my editorial was actually published, President Reagan had long stopped using the "over my dead body" phrase when asked about pulling his nominee's name, and the full Senate had rejected the Bork nomination 58 to 42.

Along with covering the White House for Fox, I had also been given the opportunity to fill in for my mentor Brit Hume as substitute anchor for *Special Report* on Friday nights. Anchoring and field reporting are two completely different animals, so hosting Brit's show was a lot of fun and a wonderful opportunity for me.

I was also anchoring on the weekends for a Fox News show called *Weekend Live*. Pretty much working seven days a week, I was putting in a ton of hours at the network, and, like most couples, Amy and I had a running discussion about my work schedule. Despite the normal "two places at once" dilemmas all parents face, with her father's incredibly strong work ethic as a lifelong example, Amy supported me 100 percent in taking advantage of every opportunity that came my way.

There was a practical side to my work schedule as well. Paulie was just a few weeks old and not exactly pestering me every night when I came home from work to take him camping or asking me if I knew anything

about rebuilding the carburetor on a 1957 Chevy he bought online. So until he got a little older, Amy and I decided this was the perfect time in my life and career to say yes to just about every opportunity that presented itself. And I did.

Also, let's face it, the news business is the news business. News happens every hour of every day, seven days a week. It never stops. Trying to keep up with it all is sometimes like trying to take a sip of water from a full-pressured fire hose. And now with the advent of the Internet, Facebook, Twitter, e-mails, blogs, online streaming, and all the rest, the continual flow of news is at an all-time high.

But in reality, it's not just the news business. Being able to be reached anywhere on the planet every second of every day pretty much affects everyone in the workforce these days. For better or worse, with e-mail, cell phones, and texting, few people are really off the clock at 5:00 or 6:00 p.m. like they used to be, whether they're in broadcasting, banking, or bricklaying.

As a husband and father, trying to strike the proper balance between life at home and life on the job and knowing when to disconnect is something I am constantly thinking about. One of my colleagues who also thought a lot about that topic was ABC's national security correspondent, Jack McWethy. A fellow graduate of DePauw, Jack became a great friend during my time at the Pentagon, and he really went out of his way to help me when I first arrived in town.

Once, on a very long trip to Iraq, Jack and I got into a lengthy discussion about family, work, the news business, priorities, life, and just about everything else under the sun. During that conversation Jack said something to

me that I totally embraced and have tried to use in my own life ever since: "If there's one thing I can tell you, Bret, it's that as you get more and more into this day-to-day coverage and work becomes your life, just make sure when you walk through the door at home you hang up your work along with your coat. When you're at home you're at home, when you're at work, you're at work," he said. "Never confuse your career with your life. If you can do that, then you win."

I will never forget that conversation with Jack. The thing that made it such a powerful message was the fact that those were not just idle words with him. Jack lived them. Totally old-school when it came to news reporting, Jack started out in the business long before the tsunami of twenty-four-hour cable or the Internet arrived. Now that they had, he could clearly see that younger journalists coming along were going to have a much tougher time than he did to maintain and nurture family relationships in the midst of the nonstop gears of the news business. Jack somehow figured out a way to keep those gears from chewing him up. Despite the fact that I seldom wore one, I think a lot about what I affectionately call Jack's "trench-coat sermon" to me during that long trip to Iraq.

With Paulie at home recovering and me back on the job at the White House, Amy and I were both feeling pretty good, even confident, about our roles as parents and finding the proper balance in our lives. I knew we were far from being out of the woods with Paulie's heart issues, but at least we had a sense things were on track and everyone in the family was recovering and becoming better equipped to deal with whatever might come our way over the next few years.

One Friday in the middle of August, just a few weeks after Paulie had come home from the hospital, I was in the Fox bureau getting ready for *Special Report* when I got a call from Amy. Even though I was in the middle of a very hectic day and the clock was quickly marching toward 6:00 p.m., I was happy to take the call. Amy had taken Paulie to Children's for his checkup earlier in the day, and I was eager to find out how things went and also hear what ideas the doctors had about Paulie keeping his food down.

Once I got on the phone, by the background noise I could hear on the other end of the line, I knew instantly that Amy was still at Children's several hours after she should have returned home.

"Why are you still at the hospital?" I immediately asked.

"Don't get scared," Amy said, which, of course, instantly scared me to death.

"Paulie has to have surgery tomorrow," Amy said.

"What!!?"

"Don't get mad," Amy said, "but Paulie has to have surgery on his stomach."

I was completely dumbfounded by what I was hearing.

"We just can't have surgery every other day," I blurted out. "We were just in the hospital for twenty-one days. Surgery is not the answer for everything," I yelled into the phone. My mind was racing. "This makes no sense at all! Paulie has heart issues—he doesn't need surgery on his stomach! He's just having a little trouble keeping his food down, for God's sake. Those people at Children's need to take a chill pill. The surgeons over there must walk around with scalpels in their holsters like gun-

slingers itching for a fight in the old west, just looking for people to operate on!"

Knowing I was in final preparations for *Special Report*, Amy tried to stay as calm as possible and keep me from going completely nuts, which, of course, I absolutely was. Wisely, she put Dr. Kurt Newman on the phone to fill me in on what was going on with Paulie's stomach. Totally unrelated to his heart issues, Paulie had something Dr. Newman called a "pyloric stenosis" that could only be dealt with surgically. Paulie's stomach was sort of kinked up with a spasm, which explained the projectiles speeding toward us like we were facing Roger Federer at the U.S. Open. Sitting at my desk in the Fox bureau, my eyes shot skyward as I muttered to no one in particular, "Can't we just catch some kind of break here?"

I immediately asked Dr. Newman how the stomach surgery was going to affect Paulie's heart. He assured me this was a completely separate issue and a quite common surgery that shouldn't pose a problem for Paulie's recovery from his open-heart operation. After I settled down a bit, I was thankful once again that they had diagnosed Paulie's stomach issue there in the hospital and we wouldn't be racing through the streets of D.C. headed to the ER in the middle of the night.

Dr. Newman said Paulie needed to stay overnight at Children's, and the operation would be performed as soon as tomorrow. Just a few days in recovery, then he would be home, he promised. I considered asking Dr. Newman if he would put that in writing, but I didn't want him to get the idea I was an erratic and crazed parent desperately at the end of my rope.

As it happened, Amy's mom was in town, and suddenly it was like old home week at Children's for the

Baier family. All the same nurses were there, and they immediately sprang into action getting Amy diapers for Paulie and the breast pump all set up for her. Same intensive care unit. Same anesthesiologist. Hugs. Greetings. The Baiers were back! Soon I would be staring at those monitors, those same monitors at all hours of the night, I just knew it.

There is no way I could possibly increase the number of prayers I was already lofting heavenward for Paulie on a daily basis. The only thing I could figure was that I must have been slacking off in the wood-knocking department.

❋

With one open-heart surgery, one stomach surgery, and one angioplasty behind him, seven-month-old Paulie was now scheduled to have his second angioplasty in late January of 2008. Catheterizations and angioplasties were complicated enough, but they are not as invasive as full-blown open-heart operations. I was not exactly clear what the doctors were doing when they went into Paulie's arteries, but it had something to do with measuring the pressures in and around his heart.

The only analogy I could think of is when they send those hurricane hunter C-17s directly into a raging storm while it is still over the ocean to get the most accurate barometric pressure and wind speed readings possible so they know exactly what we are up against when hurricane Whoever finally comes ashore. In a sense, the doctors needed to fly directly into Paulie's artery system to get firsthand, accurate readings so they would know precisely what was going on with his heart

and give the doctors a better idea when he would need to have his next open heart–operation.

Seven months to the day he was born, Paulie was back at Children's National Medical Center.

January 31, 2008, 5:41 PM, Friday
Subject: Paul's prognosis

All of you asked for a report on what the doctor did today and what lies ahead for Paul. So here it is.

Today, Dr. Michael Slack went into Paulie's heart with a catheter (through his femoral artery in his groin) and measured all of the pressures in various spots inside his heart and in the arteries around it, including the aorta, which was the focus of the last catheterization when Dr. Slack ballooned that to open it up in December.

Dr. Slack found that the aortic arch, which had closed significantly before, was almost as open as it was when he did the last balloon, meaning that the aorta held its shape and didn't get smaller. Translation: the last angioplasty/balloon worked.

Paul's pulmonary artery, however, has narrowed. It was narrow to begin with, and because of some scarring from the original surgery, it was even narrower today. That, added to the fact that the connector, also known as a homograph (the donor baby aorta that was used to connect Paul's right ventricle to his pulmonary artery) is small to begin with. It was put in small so that it could fit behind tiny baby Paul's chest—but now 19.5 lb. Paulie has a lot more room and a lot more blood pumping through his bigger body.

The original connector also had some scarring around it and therefore is narrowed at the T. Imagine a T intersection. The pulmonary artery is the street running east to west and the connector, or homograph, is the street running north to south that Ts into the pulmonary artery. Now imagine that the streets are all supposed to be two-lane streets but in Paul's case—at that intersection—they squeeze to one lane, and even half of a lane. Cars (the blood) have a hard time getting through.

Okay, there's one analogy. Hang with me here. Because there is a traffic jam at that intersection, the right ventricle of the heart has to work extra hard to pump the blood through that area to get it to the pulmonary artery and then out to the lungs for oxygen. Dr. Slack says the energy the right ventricle uses is like expending energy to suck a milk shake through a coffee straw—it takes a lot. But in the heart's case, turn it around; the heart is pushing the blood milk shake through the coffee straw—which is Paul's connector.

The normal pressure in the right ventricle should be at about 25–28% of the left ventricle. That's normal. Paul's was measured today at 115%. That's bad. It means his right ventricle is working super hard and if left like that for an extended period of time it would fail.

Today, with the ballooning that Dr. Slack did (putting balloons in various arteries and even in the homograph and pumping them up to push back scar tissue and to widen the areas as much as possible), the pressure dropped to 60% in the right ventricle. Much better. But it won't last long. As Paulie continues to grow, he will need a new connector—a four-lane street instead of a one- or two-lane street—into

that T intersection (or a big McDonalds straw instead of the coffee straw, if you like that analogy better) to get that blood moving and to reduce the pressure in his right ventricle and on his heart overall.

In addition to that, today's catheterization found something else: what's called a pseudo aneurysm in his pulmonary artery. This happened because the pressure built up in his right ventricle—to pump that blood through the small space—then the lining of the pulmonary artery where the connector is attached (sewn in there by Dr. Jonas in the original surgery) became weak. And a bubble formed, bulging out of the artery itself like you would see with an inner tube that doesn't hold its shape.

Now—there is NOT a realistic risk that the aneurysm will rupture. BUT it needs to be dealt with fairly soon in another surgery, the same surgery where the new connector will be sewn in. (In addition to the new connector, now Dr. Jonas will have to fix the aneurysm by repairing that part of the pulmonary artery.)

Watching the pressure will determine when Paul needs to get the next surgery done. They want to wait as long as they can so that he can continue to grow and they can put the biggest possible connector in there. Ideally, they want to put in something that will take Paul to his early teenage years before he'd have to get an adult one put in.

So when the pressure reaches 100%, it's time. Again, today it's 60%. That could happen in one month. It could happen in five months. But it's gonna happen before he's one year old. And they'll be able to monitor the pressure

through the echocardiograms that Paulie has done at the cardiologist's every week or two now.

The good part: he's growing and he's thriving, both cognitively and in all growth percentiles. Also good, that we're in great hands at Children's. Dr. Slack is really one of the best in his field of catheterizations. Also good. One could argue that it's better to get this done while Paulie's very young so that he doesn't remember it when he has to do it when he's 13 or 14.

The tough part: it's been a string of tough things to have to go through with Paul early on in life. Nothing was tougher than the first surgery. The thought of having to go through another open-heart surgery with a little boy who knows his mom and dad and smiles all the time and who you hate to see upset in any way, shape, or form—and who has been through so much already—makes us sick to our stomachs, literally. But it's what we have to do. And one day, we'll look back on this time as a flash. But right now it seems very unfair. It will be very difficult—extremely—because, to be honest with you, this catheterization today was not easy. It is, however, the hand we've been dealt, and we think the guy upstairs has us covered.

That's the long and the short of it. Doctors say that if all goes well, Paulie can live a long and almost completely normal life (minus the occasional cardiologist appointment). So—once we get through the next big surgery (in one to five months) there will likely be a few more catheterization lab appointments. But the idea is to get the catheterizations to about one every five years. And then ideally we'd have only one more surgery after that when he's 13 or so.

*That's where we are. Thanks for all the support and love
and prayers.*

Love you all,
Bret and Amy

When he was almost eight months old, and with his
rookie year stat sheet now filled up with two angioplasties, two surgeries, and another heart surgery scheduled
in a few short months, Amy and I were completely
amazed at how resilient—even strong—Paulie seemed
to be. As inspiring as his resilience and warrior strength
were to everyone who came in contact with him, that
was also part of his problem.

Paulie was growing so fast, the donated aorta he had
in his body couldn't grow along with the rest of him.
He would need the second heart operation so he could
get a new homograph put in to keep up with his growing body. There are hopes that one day replacing those
connectors might be done by going through the arteries
just like an angioplasty, but for now, surgery through
the chest wall is the only way the replacement can take
place.

Watching Paulie through the winter months of 2007
and into 2008, I was amazed at everything he had endured before he ever reached his first birthday. At eight
months old, our little fighter had certainly experienced
enough trauma and excitement for a lifetime. If we
could just get Paulie through the next heart surgery and
to his first birthday and then to the place where we
could have a solid four- to five-year stretch of catheter-

izations and angioplasties and no surgeries for a while, you would probably find me doing cartwheels out on the National Mall all the way from the Washington Monument to the Capitol.

"Sometimes the end comes like a thief in the night."

Those words came from Sam Donaldson, and unfortunately, Sam was not unleashing a snarky metaphor at the president in the Rose Garden about a failed nomination or doomed piece of legislation on Capitol Hill. Sam was solemnly quoting from the Bible as his voice echoed throughout the auditorium of the Newseum just a few blocks from the United States Capitol.

Sam was onstage delivering one of many tributes to our friend and colleague John McWethy. One week earlier, Jack, just sixty years old, had died in a skiing accident in Colorado where he had recently retired with his wife, Laurie. I, along with everyone else gathered to pay respects, was extremely sad about the loss of our beloved colleague and friend who had been such a huge influence on so many of us in and out of the news business.

I had so many great memories of Jack: working as competitors side by side at the Pentagon, taking trips together to Afghanistan and Iraq, and, of course, our mutual love of golf. As I sat in that memorial service and heard all those tributes for my friend, my mind was racing with thoughts about life and death, the fragile line dividing the two, the brevity of it all, and being someone like Jack who made a real difference in this world, not only through the words he spoke but by the way he lived his life.

CBS News national security correspondent David Martin spoke about the day Jack retired and how he felt like the guy in the Paul Simon song who asks, "Who will be my role model now that my role model is gone?" That's exactly how I felt. Jack not only set the standard for being a dogged, fearless reporter, he did it with integrity, class, and great humor. But beyond that, Jack figured out how to compete at the highest levels of the nation's journalistic stage without becoming mean-spirited or taking shortcuts, all the while keeping his family life front and center. That is one serious accomplishment.

After the service I went up to Jack's wife, Laurie, and told her about the great influence Jack had on me and specifically about the trench-coat sermon he delivered to me on that flight to Iraq just a few years before. When I recounted the story, Laurie said, "That's exactly how Jack lived his life."

Sam Donaldson's quote about the end sometimes coming like a thief in the night really got me thinking. What a great example Jack had been, not only in journalism but in life itself. I wondered if I would ever come close to having the same kind of impact on people's lives that Jack did. I left the Newseum that day with a new sense of urgency, not about my career in journalism but more fundamentally about the kind of person I wanted to be with whatever time the Lord gave me here on this earth.

Walking along Pennsylvania Avenue after the service and thinking about the example Jack had been for us all, I wondered what kind of example I was for people around me, for my wife and my son—especially for a son who was setting the bar extremely high in the area

of courage and inspiration. While my career was firing on all cylinders and Amy was extremely supportive of all the time I was spending on the job, Jack's trench coat at the door story was reverberating through my mind as I walked. Time is so precious, and unfortunately it can take something like a memorial service or a funeral to wake us up to that fact. I wasn't wearing a coat that day, but when I got home later that evening I made a special point of hanging my day job up by the door as I walked in. Hugging my wife and son a little harder than normal, I reflected on all the challenges of the past eight months. Taking nothing for granted, I thanked God for every precious moment he had allowed us to share together and for the daily miracle of grace and strength he had given us to carry on.

CHAPTER NINE

To Whom Much Is Given

For those following presidential politics, 2008 was turning out to be one incredibly interesting news year.

After his campaign implosion the previous summer, then being written off as political roadkill by the pundits and prognosticators, Arizona senator John McCain fought his way to the front of the pack in the race for the GOP nomination. On the other side of the aisle, charismatic first-term senator Barack Obama of Illinois, with record crowds and seemingly bottomless coffers of campaign cash, was completely discombobulating former first lady and New York senator Hillary Clinton's plans to capture the Democratic nomination. With home mortgages melting down from coast to coast, the financial crisis on Wall Street, and the U.S. economy teetering on the brink, no matter how the presidential race turned out, 2008 promised to be a memorable year for news—one for the record books.

On the nonpresidential front, 2008 was turning out to be quite a memorable year for the Baier family, too. On April 29, Paulie was scheduled to return to Children's National Medical Center for his second open-heart surgery, ten months to the day he was born. To keep up with Paulie's growing body, Dr. Richard Jonas needed to go back in so he could swap the baby aorta he put in the previous July for a larger one. Despite all his time in the hospital, medical procedures, surgeries, and the general fragility of his heart and arteries, little Paulie was becoming quite a big boy these days, weighing in at almost twenty-three pounds.

In fact, Paulie's rapid growth was the reason he needed the second operation so soon. During the previous summer's first open-heart operation, Paulie's tiny chest cavity pretty much dictated the size of the original homograph connector Dr. Jonas was able to graft in. Now that Paulie was growing so big so fast, that original connector was starting to leak and needed to be replaced with a larger one. There was, however, an upside to all of Paulie's rapid growth. With the extra room in his chest cavity, Dr. Jonas might now be able to graft in a larger connector than he had originally anticipated.

Although it was a foregone conclusion that the first homograph would eventually fail and have to come out, without jeopardizing Paulie's health the doctors wanted to hold off as long as possible before scheduling the surgery so they could put in the largest connector possible and create as much space on the calendar between this surgery and the next.

No matter what size homograph they would be able to fit in Paulie's chest, there was no doubt he would still need to undergo several catheterizations and angioplasties over the next few years in order to keep his arteries open and flowing. Although angioplasties are not exactly a walk in the park, I would take a hundred of them over one open-heart surgery any day of the week. And by the way things seemed to be going for us, we might just hit that one hundred number before all was said and done.

Despite our nervousness about the upcoming operation, Amy and I were trying to enjoy every precious moment we had with Paulie at home. Heart issues aside, we were really getting a kick out of watching our little man as he discovered the big wide world around him. Even with all the challenges in his young life, Paulie was turning out to be quite a boy's boy, exploring every nook and cranny around the condo and showing extreme curiosity about each new discovery, especially dogs, birds, and the boats on the Potomac River.

Paulie was crawling everywhere and conquering every obstacle that had the audacity to block him from wherever his expeditionary spirit told him he needed to go. One of his favorite activities lately was walking behind his Winnie the Pooh train as he pushed it around the condo. Paulie was also developing a distinct personality. With Amy and me both card-carrying members of the type A personality club, it didn't shock either of us that our son hit the genetic jackpot in the strong will department. Paulie was very adorable, very sweet—but *very* strong willed. Amy and I spent a fair amount of time discussing just whose particular gene pool might have fueled the latest record-setting decibels coming out of that little body.

Because I was a good match for him, just a day or two before the surgery I went into the hospital and gave blood that could be used during the upcoming operation. Somewhere in the middle of squeezing that ball they give you to make the blood flow faster and then seeing it rush into the bag, it hit me that this second open-heart surgery was really upon us. We, of course, knew Dr. Jonas was the best in his field and the quality of the care at Children's National Medical Center was second to none. But still, twenty-three pounds or not, I was constantly worrying about just how much trauma Paulie's body could take before he even reached his first birthday.

Even though we knew a new homograph connector would buy Paulie several more years before he would need another operation, as the actual day approached, Amy and I grew more and more anxious about going through all this one more time. We were both extremely agitated and having a tough time in our own ways. Amy was experiencing really bad migraine headaches, and I was having a lot of difficulty sleeping.

Just a few days before the surgery I was walking on Pennsylvania Avenue right in front of the White House when I saw a woman coming toward me toting a big cardboard display of one kind or another. About a half block away, I couldn't make out what it was she was carrying. But as she got closer I could see she was holding an oversize cardboard replica of the front cover of the popular Top Doctors Issue of *Washingtonian Magazine*.

· On the magazine cover seen on the poster was Paulie's surgeon, Dr. Richard Jonas. The woman told me her mother was also listed in the issue, and she had asked the bookstore near the White House if she could have the display when they were done with it.

When I got home later that night, I told Amy about the woman with the poster of Dr. Jonas. Like me, she got very excited about another one of those chance encounters that seemed to be there for us whenever

our troubled spirits needed it most. And we definitely needed it that week. Whether pure coincidence or a re-inforcing bit of encouragement from above to remind us we were on the right path, it didn't really matter to me one way or the other. Amy and I both slept just a little bit better that night.

❦

April 29, 2008, 6:32 PM, Tuesday
Subject: Thank you—so far so good

Thank you all for your prayers, your thoughts, and your good wishes. Paul is now in the Cardiac Intensive Care Unit at Children's recovering from what his surgeon is calling a very successful open-heart surgery. While Paul is just start-ing to wake up (opening his eyes for a few minutes at a time), his vital signs all look very good so far.

Late this afternoon, the doctors took out his breathing tube, which is a huge development this early, and his parents are cautiously breathing a big sigh of relief. While there will be some long days ahead in the hospital, his doctors say the prognosis looks very good, and (knock on wood) we could be home in five to six days, which would be ahead of the predicted schedule.

An early morning started at 5:00 a.m., and because Paul couldn't eat or drink anything from midnight until the surgery at 7:30 a.m., we expected him to be cranky. But he wasn't. He was actually in a very good mood and was literally crawl-ing all over the bed in the pre-op area and even chomping on his hospital gown ties (he WAS hungry, after all).

As Mom and Dad were increasingly anxious, Paul didn't have a care in the world besides trying to play the bed like a drum every few minutes. Even when the anesthesiologist came to take him to surgery already wearing her mask, Paulie pointed to her mask with his finger as he went to her. We reluctantly handed him over, squeezing and kissing him a few more times. As they carried him down the hall away from us to go to the operating room, that's when we could hear him start to cry, leaving his two parents in a pre-op room to shed a tear or two as well.

During surgery parents are given pagers to be updated throughout. The wait is the excruciating thing, so any blip of information is like gold.

8:55 a.m. the pager buzzed: "First chest incision just took place."

9:41 a.m.: "Paul is now on bypass" (the heart-lung machine that essentially takes over for his heart as the surgery takes place).

And then for an hour, complete pager silence.

Trying to read the newspaper is not possible without constantly glancing down to make sure the pager on your belt is working. We knew the surgery was supposed to last four to five hours—this was going to be the longest and toughest part. But then, suddenly, a buzz from the belt, and I almost spit out my Diet Coke.

10:45 a.m.: "Paul is off bypass and Dr. Jonas will see you soon in the waiting room."

The surgery was over much sooner than we expected. After 20 more minutes that felt like 55, Dr. Jonas came into the waiting room and smiled, saying in his Australian accent, "All went very well." The homograph (the conduit that Paulie had replaced that connects his right ventricle to his pulmonary artery) fit well, and Dr. Jonas repaired the area (aneurysm) that needed to be fixed.

Imagine sewing a donated baby aorta (a very small piece of a donor baby's organ) onto a walnut-size heart that is still beating as you are sewing, using minuscule stitches to patch an area where my son's blood flows to keep him alive. It boggles the mind. Dr. Jonas truly is a gifted man, and we are extremely fortunate to have him as Paulie's surgeon. We have some hurdles to cross in recovery, but we believe Paul is a true fighter and he'll be back crawling and walking behind his Winnie the Pooh train in no time!

We just found out that we can actually thank the family who donated the baby aorta through the Washington Regional Transplant Consortium (WRTC). However, the consortium only allows you to do it anonymously. There are now two families that have helped Paulie live. WRTC has a printed note that recipients can then attach to a personalized message. The WRTC then sends the note to the donor families.

Here's how it reads:

"The spirit of gratitude knows no season, it only knows of kindness and of love. Every day throughout the year, you have my sincere gratitude for giving me the opportunity of renewed life, a priceless gift of hope through organ dona-

tion. May you always find comfort and peace with the gift you have given. I am forever grateful!"

We will now write two notes on Paulie's behalf and have them sent to the donor families—to whom we are eternally grateful. As we walk through Children's we realize how many grateful families come out of here each week. The doctors and nurses do amazing work to try to get and keep kids healthy.

Thank you all again. We are now on the right track to getting home. The power of the prayers and the good thoughts really helped us through again, and they're really helping Paulie bounce back fast. We come away again only appreciating life more and acknowledging how important every minute with family can be.

Sincerely,
Bret and Amy

A few days after his second open-heart surgery in ten months, I decided to update everyone on the progress Paulie was making as he recuperated at home. I was hoping this would be my last communication about Paulie's health for a good long while. I prayed we were about to enter an uneventful period of calm and normalcy with no medical news to report for at least four or five years.

May 4, 2008, 8:08 PM, Sunday
Subject: Back on the train!

Thank you all for your prayers and good wishes—we believe they paid off. Paul is home, he's on the mend in his

own environment, and he is thriving. It has been quite a week of worrying during some long, sleepless nights at Children's, but he did it again. He came through his second open-heart surgery like a champ.

All of the wires and tubes attached to him were making Paulie pretty upset. I would be, too! To go from crawling with toys in your home to being connected to tubes and wires and an oxygen tank—no, thank you! At times Amy was allowed to crawl into the bed with Paul to try to calm him down.

Staying with Paul in a room on the heart and kidney floor at Children's there were some scary times (hence the e-mail silence). Paulie had a fever that he eventually fought off. But the scare of infection was real (and that's what docs are most concerned about postsurgery).

In addition, Paul was clearly in pain a few times and very uncomfortable. The grimace turned to a whimper turned to an all-out cry is a tough progression to watch for any parent. The whole thing was a much different experience this time. Paul's now a big boy who is used to being mobile, yet he still can't talk to tell us what hurts or what he needs. While he was really out of it and wiped out the first two days, he quickly came back to his old smiling self on day three.

We are always amazed at how resilient kids are. But once you go through two heart surgeries, "resilient" really doesn't do it justice. We always remember that he couldn't bounce back without the work of his amazing surgeon and the doctors and nurses who work with him. Dr. Jonas and his team

are truly remarkable—we can't say enough about them and what they do.

Paul was in a great mood when we found out we were going home. It's like he knew what the doctors were saying and he couldn't stop smiling. His Mom and Dad were a little wiped out from alternating overnight stays at Paulie's cribside. But Paul's grandparents are in town to help keep him in good spirits.

The bottom line is this—the surgery was a success. So far, the recovery is going amazingly well and remarkably fast (even faster than last time). And Paul's first order of business when we got home—you guessed it—that Winnie the Pooh train. At first, we were very worried about his movement. But the doctors say he will self-regulate and he will determine what he can and can't do. They told us to let him explore. He now walks behind that Winnie the Pooh train with a new chest scar barely peeking through his shirt—it's the most beautiful chest scar we've ever seen.

I hope not to "reply to all" for quite some time. But thank you ALL for your prayers and good wishes. We believe the Big Guy upstairs must have some big things in store for Paulie. We are just along for his train ride.

Sincerely,
Bret and Amy

Sunday, June 29, 2008, brought joy and rejoicing throughout the Baier home in Georgetown. Paul Fran-

cis "Paulie" Baier had done it. One year old! Two open-heart operations, one stomach surgery, and two angioplasties: Paulie was a living, breathing one-year-old miracle and an honest-to-God example of resilience, grit, stamina, heart, and determination. And he was my son! I couldn't have been more proud of him for the way he endured—even triumphed—over everything that came his way during his extremely challenging first year of life.

The doctors were fairly confident the new donated baby aorta now in Paulie's chest would last him a good five or six years. And although he would definitely need several more procedures before he entered kindergarten, for the first time in a long time Amy and I felt hope for the future. We could begin to see a clear path for Paulie having as much of a normal little-boy life as possible: romping around the condo, hikes with Mom and Dad down by the river, holidays with our families, trips to the park, first day at school, playdates with the other kids—and especially walking on the golf course with his dad on a cool autumn day.

On the heels of Paulie's first birthday, Saturday, July 12, 2008, promised to be another day of great celebration and joy around the Baier house. As it was one year to the day when Paulie underwent his first lifesaving open-heart operation, we considered this to be the anniversary of the day we were given a second chance with our precious son.

Sadly, July 12 was also the day we received news that my friend and colleague Tony Snow had died of cancer at the age of fifty-three. Less than a year ago Tony stood at the White House briefing room podium and welcomed me back after Paulie's first surgery. Just a few

months before that, he had returned to the briefing room after being away for five weeks of chemotherapy. Tony stood tall at the podium that day, telling us all "I am a very lucky guy" and "You've got to realize you've got the gift of life. So make the most of it." What an amazing spirit Tony had. And now he was gone.

Unlike Jack McWethy's unanticipated death just a few months before, most of us who knew Tony suspected his courageous battle was coming to an end. That didn't make the news any easier. To be sure, it was a blessing that Tony was no longer suffering. But the reality that his bright light and overflowing spirit were now gone from this world was hard to grasp.

Tony had left his White House post late the previous year and had taken a new job as a commentator for CNN. So over the past few years I had known Tony as a colleague at Fox News, an adversary in the White House briefing room, and most recently as a competitor at CNN. But no matter where he happened to be working, Tony was always a joy and delight to know and truly a gentleman. Later that day, on Fox News Channel's *Weekend Live*, I paid tribute to him by going on air and reading in his honor "The True Gentleman," by John Walter Wayland:

> The True Gentleman is a man whose conduct proceeds from good will and an acute sense of propriety, and whose self-control is equal to all emergencies; who does not make the poor man conscious of his poverty, the obscure man of his obscurity, or any man of his inferiority or deformity; who is himself humbled when necessity compels him to humble another; who does not

flatter wealth, cringe before power, or boast of his own possessions or achievements; who speaks with frankness but with sincerity and sympathy always; whose deed follows his word; who thinks of the rights and feelings of others rather than his own; and who appears well in any company, a man with whom honor is sacred and virtue is safe.

In his homily at Tony's funeral at the Basilica at Catholic University, university president David M. O'Connell seemed to capture perfectly the essence of Tony's life when he said, "The measure of this man's life can be found in his character, in his optimism, in his joy and humor, in his courage, in his passion for what was good and right, and in his love for God and family and neighbor and country. Tony Snow did not need a long life for us to measure. It was, rather, we who needed his life to be longer."

It was difficult to comprehend. During the 2008 presidential campaign and in the midst of this absolute monster of a news year in American politics, along with Jack McWethy and Tony Snow, longtime *Meet the Press* anchor Tim Russert died of a heart attack while at the NBC bureau in Washington, D.C.

Although I didn't know Tim as well as I knew Tony or Jack, he was someone I always looked up to personally and professionally. Tim was probably the best American television news interviewer of his generation. No one could grill a public official trying to hold something back better than Tim Russert.

Once on a campaign trip I found myself talking to Tim about everything—sports, religion, politics, and, of course, the art of interviewing. I remember Tim telling

me that the absolute best quality of a good interviewer was the ability to listen to your guest and not be so infatuated with all the brilliant questions you have jotted down on your three-by-five cards. Perhaps not the most keen theological observation ever, but the only thing I could figure was that the Lord himself had taken some kind of personal interest in the American political scene in 2008 and decided to recruit Jack, Tony, and Tim for his own all-star panel.

The rest of 2008 was unbelievably busy for everyone working in the news business. And like every other journalist in town, I was up to my eyeballs in assignments. Along with covering the final year of the George W. Bush presidency, I was still anchoring *Special Report* on Friday nights; a two-hour show, *Weekend Live*; and a political analysis show called *The Strategy Room* on Sunday nights. I also served as a floor reporter for the political conventions in Denver and Minneapolis that summer. As news years go, 2008 was at the top of the heap, and I was privileged to be in the middle of all the action.

I always knew I wanted to be a journalist. The news business is intensely competitive, and to pursue it professionally you need to have your eyes wide open and develop a very thick skin early on. I had received great training at DePauw University, was always a pretty decent writer, was curious about everything and smart enough, I suppose. But, as in a lot of professions, there are always smarter, better-looking, or better-whatever folks around who think they can do the job as well as you can.

That said, although I never felt I was the best-looking, the smartest, or the best whatever in the room, I always felt as if I had a secret weapon, if you could call it that.

On any job I was ever given, I simply refused to allow myself to be outworked by anyone. And that attitude and work ethic seemed to be appreciated by my bosses over the years.

Going back to my first days in the Atlanta bureau, to the Pentagon, the White House, and now the 2008 presidential election, Fox had given me more once-in-a-lifetime opportunities than I could ever count. Over the past ten years I had traveled to seventy-four countries, taking trips with defense secretaries, generals, the vice president, and the president of the United States on Air Force One. In addition to my personal home life with Paulie and Amy, I felt that I had found my professional home at Fox. The way I showed my gratitude for all the opportunities that came to me over the years was to never be a clock-watcher and always work until the job was done. If that approach to my work happened to be rewarded with a front-row seat to history, that was okay, too. And boy, 2008 was quite a year to have a front-row seat.

No matter where you happened to be on the political spectrum, the election of Illinois senator Barack Obama as the nation's first-ever African American president was a moment to remember. The fact that an African American was going to stand on the steps of the slave-built Capitol, left hand on the Bible and his right raised to take the presidential oath—now that was going to be a true American moment. Like I said—what a year to have a front-row seat!

Apart from all the political news of 2008, what an amazing, life-affirming, and perspective-altering year it had been for Amy and me! Watching our courageous son triumphantly emerge from his surgeries and hospi-

talizations over the past year not only deepened us as individuals but also forced us to start rethinking our priorities.

It's funny in a way. Before Paulie was born, Amy and I would take our evening walks around Georgetown and talk about our hopes and dreams for the future, our family, how many children we wanted to have, how we wanted to make a difference with our lives, and all the other things excited young couples talk about as they start to carve their path.

On one particular evening walk just a few weeks before Paulie was born, we were discussing specific charities we might want to be involved with in the D.C. area. With its politicians, VIPs, and movers and shakers of all stripes, Washington is a very social town with multiple black-tie charity events that one can go to pretty much every night of the week. Apart from the impracticality of attending events every night, and despite the worthiness of so many of the causes, Amy and I talked a lot about which organizations we might devote ourselves to so we could make a difference beyond simply attending black-tie fund-raisers, as important as they are.

Amy and I grew up in families in which giving back and paying it forward were high on the priority list. Both of our families believed strongly in the words of Jesus, "To whom much is given, of him will much be required." Even before Paulie came along, Amy and I considered ourselves to be extremely blessed people, especially being born in the country we were born in and that God had placed us in the families he did. From a young age we were both taught that charity, generosity, and looking after those who need a helping hand is the secret to living a meaningful and virtuous life.

Amy's father, Paul Francis Hills, a very successful businessman in Chicago, and her mother, Barbie Hills, are off the charts when it comes to philanthropy and generosity, and they infused Amy with that same spirit of giving. When we were young boys growing up in the suburbs of Atlanta, my mother used to take my brother and me to downtown soup kitchens so we would have a firsthand lesson in the truth that "There, but for the grace of God, go I." From the earliest days of our relationship, Amy and I connected on being concerned about others and giving back to the community, and we wanted to continue to build on this tradition in our own family.

In addition to the great influence of families, friends, churches, and communities, I have often been struck by the role that unscripted—even nondescript—conversations, encounters, or experiences can play in helping shape the direction one's life might eventually take. It might start out as something quite small, even seemingly insignificant: a quick conversation at a gas pump with a complete stranger, something you see on a billboard, a lyric from a song, a homily at church, or any one of the thousands of other chance encounters we have during our lifetimes.

No matter how it happens, something from that experience or encounter, perhaps unnoticed at the time, takes root in your heart and mind and begins to grow. Then, in due season, before you even know it, that original and seemingly insignificant seed has miraculously blossomed to the point where it becomes a major part of your life. I can identify a few of those unscripted moments, those planted seeds, in my own life that took root and started to give me a vision for how I might one day make a difference for good in this world.

One was on Thanksgiving Day in 1994.

Just two years out of college, I was living in Washington, D.C., tending bar, looking for a job in television, and dreaming of the day when I might make my mark in journalism. My mother had come to visit me during the holidays, and instead of having our own Thanksgiving dinner or going out to a fancy restaurant, we decided to spend the day volunteering at a local soup kitchen.

When we arrived at the soup kitchen early in the morning, we quickly discovered that the operation, as good-hearted as it was, was completely disorganized. To help out a bit and improve the situation, I informally started organizing some of the other lost volunteers who were there to help but were being given no guidance of any kind.

I looked around the room and started suggesting to folks what they might do to help: "Why don't you do the pies? How about peas and carrots for you? You wanna do the turkey?"

Nobody gave me any kind of authority. I just decided to fill the leadership void of the moment until someone else showed up to take over. My mom and I were just like everyone else at the soup kitchen, simply wanting to volunteer and give back on this great day of thanks. But with no one around to tell us what to do, we just started doing.

The plan for the day, apparently, was to get all this food organized, cooked, packed up, and driven a few blocks away to the grounds of the U.S. Capitol, where it would be served on folding tables to whomever showed up and needed a meal. As more and more volunteers started arriving at the soup kitchen, folks started coming up to me and asking, "What do you

want me to do?" It wasn't long before even the guy in charge of the soup kitchen that day was asking me what I wanted him to do.

Eventually I took a roll call of all the volunteers to see who had transportation so we could come up with a plan to transport the food up to the Capitol in time for the promised noontime meal. Soon, all the volunteers, including my mom and me, found ourselves on the Capitol lawn serving Thanksgiving dinner to a very long line of some very grateful folks happy to have a hot meal on this day of thanks.

As I was standing at one of the tables serving up turkey and my mom was down the line on the peas, I looked up and saw that several local TV crews had arrived to do a story on all these folks being fed at the Capitol. Soon, one of the volunteers tapped me on the shoulder and told me "they"—the TV people—"want to talk to the person in charge": *me!*

No one else really wanted to do it, so over the next thirty minutes I did several television interviews for the local stations, explaining what was going on right there in the shadow of the glorious dome of the Capitol.

It wasn't exactly like I was looking for any kind of fame or fortune when I woke up that morning. Mom and I simply wanted to do something—anything—on the spur of the moment to volunteer and give back on Thanksgiving Day.

I had to laugh. I couldn't get my foot in the door at any of the television stations that were now interviewing me and putting me on their evening newscasts. But there I was, part-time bartender/aspiring television reporter Bret Baier, being interviewed by the top stations in the D.C. market. I wound up on the news in Wash-

ington after all. Later in the evening, when we returned home, my roommates were absolutely amazed: "What happened? We thought you were going up there to volunteer and hand out turkey to some homeless people. We've been watching you on TV all afternoon doing interviews like you were the mayor or something!"

That experience got me thinking not only about leadership, or sometimes the lack of it, but also that sometimes the dividing line between success and failure for a project is simply one person stepping in to fill the gap and putting themselves in the uncomfortable position of speaking up or even taking charge, if that is required. Without my mother's influence in my life, I doubt I would have ever suggested volunteering that day, let alone assumed any kind of leadership role to get those people fed. But once my mother and I were there, we were on the job and we were all in.

Another one of those unscripted moments that had a big effect on me over the years came during my first full year in Washington. Early in 2002, after I had only been in town for a few months and was covering the Pentagon, if I had any kind of hangout at all it was Cafe Milano, an upscale restaurant and bar in Georgetown. It was and still is a great place to meet with sources, make new contacts, and generally pick up on the political buzz of the town.

I was a young reporter looking to meet folks, make connections, and learn all I could about the politics of the town, the Pentagon, defense spending, and anything else I could pick up along the way. Lots of movers and shakers hung out at Cafe Milano, and being the new kid in town, I figured it was going to be my place, too.

One night there I happened to meet a guy named Joe

Robert. Being new in town I really didn't know much about Joe, but he was a Fox watcher and knew I covered the Pentagon for the network. Joe and I started having really interesting discussions about Afghanistan, Iraq, foreign affairs, and any number of other topics in the news during those days.

This was before I met Amy and when the idea of invading Iraq and toppling Saddam Hussein was just that—an idea. Joe wasn't sold on the Bush administration's view on weapons of mass destruction as it related to Iraq or the need to go after Saddam Hussein as part of the overall war on terror. Being a pragmatist, Joe also had serious concerns that we could keep the heat on al Qaeda and the Taliban in Afghanistan and go after Saddam Hussein at the same time. Joe was incredibly interested in foreign policy, but his real interest in Iraq was much more personal in nature. He was the father of a marine who would likely go to Iraq if we invaded. One night Joe told me: "I really don't want my son to go, but if he does, I'm going to support him a thousand percent. I may even go over there, too, sometime."

Working at the Pentagon for Fox, I traveled to Afghanistan and Iraq twenty-three times between 2001 and 2007, but I had never heard of a father going over to visit his son in the middle of a war zone. But sure enough, after the invasion of Iraq, Joe, indeed, made good on his promise to visit his son. I have no idea how he pulled that off, but he did. Not long after, despite his misgivings about us being in Iraq in the first place, Joe helped organize a benefit concert at Camp Pendleton, California, for the troops: Kiss, Ted Nugent, Destiny's Child, and Godsmack were just a few of the big acts Joe recruited to perform. Joe was one

of those guys who really knew how to pull strings and get things done.

When I first met Joe I didn't know much about him, but over time I learned he was a very successful businessman who had made hundreds of millions of dollars in financial services and real estate, a true American rags-to-riches story. Despite growing up very poor, as a young boy Joe had a real knack for earning money: selling newspapers, Christmas trees, applesauce, and bacon door-to-door and working in various restaurants around town.

Once as a schoolboy Joe found some boxing equipment that had been thrown away, and he used it to organize neighborhood boxing matches in his backyard, charging a fee and selling concessions. Talk about planted seeds. Later, when he had become a big success, Joe used his backyard-boxing idea as the basis for creating an annual Fight Night event in D.C. that has raised tens of millions of dollars over the years for numerous charities around town.

Joe's life was a book, a feature film, a documentary, and a graduate level course in business all rolled into one. Despite all his wealth, success, and intense interest in American politics and foreign policy, Joe and I eventually connected on a whole other level. After Paulie was born and we learned he had to have open-heart surgery, the operation was performed in the Joe Robert Surgical Center at Children's National Medical Center. The surgical center had been named for Joe after he made a sizable financial contribution to the hospital.

In 2000, Joe's son was at Children's to have surgery on his ribs, and Joe wound up sleeping on the floor to be right by his son's bed. With all the noise and general

discomfort of the situation, Joe had a very bad night. But Joe being Joe, he figured he was in a position to do something about it, so he did. That's the thing about Joe; he didn't just complain about stuff. If he was in a position to change things, he put his money where his mouth was. Joe was one of those people who knew how to go all in and make a difference for good.

In 2007, after he learned my son was in Children's for his first surgery, Joe and I reconnected, and he became a great source of personal strength and a wonderful example to me in the area of giving back and going all in to help people. My relationship with Joe had pretty much started as one of those unscripted encounters at Cafe Milano back when I first arrived in town.

Perhaps the most significant unscripted moment having to do with life priorities and making a difference was also the shortest. It was the night of June 30, 2007, just one day after Paulie was born and within the first hour of our family sojourn at Children's National Medical Center. I was standing with Amy's father, Paul Hills, at the bank of elevators as we made our way to one-day-old Paulie who had just been transferred to Children's Cardiac Intensive Care Unit. Waiting for the elevator, we were both emotionally spent. Big Paul turned to me and said, "In one way, Bret, you are very fortunate. You have found your cause. This is why people fill up all those ballrooms on Saturday night. Why guys wear tuxedos they don't want to wear and the women get all dressed up and buy auction items they don't really need. As good-hearted and generous as they are, in many cases those folks are supporting causes they know very little about. From now on, you will never be that person. You have your cause."

Paul Hills was right. Although I didn't know it at the time, the seed of an idea he planted in me during that one-minute conversation at those elevators took root and grew in me over the first year of Paulie's life.

For Amy and me, raising and nurturing our son was obviously number one in our lives. Beyond that, if we could do anything for the folks who gave us our son back, we were going to do it. Children's National Medical Center had been a blessing in our lives and gave us a second chance with our precious son. Almost as important, they gave us hope. If Amy and I could do something—anything—to help Children's offer that same kind of hope to other parents facing similar circumstances, we were all in. And God willing, when he got older, medical challenges or not, we hoped and prayed that Paulie would be standing there side by side with us, thankful for all the blessings in this life and for life itself.

Totally above and beyond any career achievements in television or journalism, if one day I was able to look up and see my son living his life to the fullest with joy and gratefulness in his heart and a spirit of helping others around him, I would count my own life a success.

❀

Apart from the big news on the American political scene, as the year 2008 drew to a close there were also a few news items right there in the Fox D.C. bureau. I learned that my mentor and friend Brit Hume decided to step away from the *Special Report* anchor desk, and Roger Ailes wanted me to take his place. Given that no one in journalism could ever take Brit Hume's place, I

was incredibly humbled by the opportunity I was being offered and the trust that Roger placed in me in asking me to take the helm of the network's flagship political show. I had no idea how things were going to turn out, but I committed myself to doing everything in my power to make sure *Special Report* was as crisp and relevant as it was the entire time Brit was at the helm.

We celebrated the start of 2009 with a trip to Naples, Florida, giving me a little time to decompress, catch my breath and reflect on everything the Baier family had experienced over the past year.

Looking back, I had to admit it seemed like a tumultuous, multicolored blur.

Somehow, through faith, prayer, and the loving support of our family and friends, we had emerged from the storm—a little banged up and scarred, perhaps, but far from broken.

Being in Florida also gave me time to consider the new opportunities and responsibilities Amy and I had been entrusted with both on the job and at home as we raised our precious son who we truly considered a miracle and gift from God.

As the celebration of the New Year began to subside and the echo of the fireworks faded, I could hear the strains of a still, small voice deep within.

At first it was nothing by a faint whisper, but eventually the familiar words grew loud, strong and clean, and I hoped I was ready for the challenge.

"To whom much is given, of him will much be required."

CHAPTER TEN

Special Heart

"Hey, Daddy, I called to say happy birthday to you. I hope you have a nice meeting with the doctor and he will help you, and I hope you have a nice time doing it. Your family is at home, and I hope you have a nicer birthday than anybody. You are the best dad in the whole entire universe, and I love you more than anything, and you are the best dad. I love you more than anything."

Not since the phone call from President Bush during Paulie's first surgery in the summer of 2007 have I been happier about missing a call and letting the message go directly to voice mail. It was August 2013, and I was at the doctor's office for a checkup when six-year-old Paulie called me to wish me happy birthday.

Paulie was becoming such a mature little man these days.

All grown up, he was helping his mom and dad around the house, watching after his little brother, Daniel, and of course borrowing Amy's cell phone from time to time to make important phone calls. Paulie's in-

tuition and growing maturity no doubt tipped him off to the fact that he was competing with a former leader of the free world in the category of electronic family keepsakes. Thirty seconds after leaving his first message, Paulie felt compelled to call back to make sure there was absolutely no confusion about who it was who placed the original call: "Hey, Daddy, this is Paul. I wanted to tell you that other message was from your son Paul, and I love you, and you are the best dad and you are awesome. You are so awesome. You're awesomer than any dad. You are nicer than any dad, and we're going to have a nice family time on your birthday, and I hope we have a nice vacation. Bye, Daddy."

These spectacular everyday vignettes presented by Paulie—and increasingly by and with Daniel—were now playing themselves out pretty much daily around the Baier home in northwest Washington. Amy and I were enthralled every time and thrilled to have our own box seats for all daily performances and especially the weekend matinees.

As much as I enjoyed anchoring Fox News Channel's *Special Report* and considered myself extremely fortunate to have a front-row seat to history and the politics of the nation, nothing from the White House or Capitol Hill could ever compete with the adrenaline rush I got whenever the stage lights went up for the latest edition of the *2013 Baier Brothers' Review*.

A few years back, to accommodate the growing Baier family, we moved out of our Georgetown condo down on the river and into a bigger house so all the Baier boys, including me, would have plenty of space for our ever-increasing arsenal of boy supplies, sports equipment, balls, plastic tractors, basketball hoops, and, of course,

our Sports Authority–scale inventory of little boy and big boy golf equipment.

Paulie and Daniel were becoming such grown-up little men lately. In fact, Paulie recently informed Amy and me that he now wanted us to start calling him Paul instead of Paulie. The request was about him feeling more like a big boy, which I immediately interpreted as having something to do with a recent playground encounter he might have had with a bigger kid previously known as Frankie, Freddie, or Willie. I suspect the newly minted Frank, Fred, or Will was probably allowed to retire his own "ie" as a birthday gift, or possibly it was part of some grand family negotiation involving a promise to put all dirty clothes in the hamper and feeding Fluffy every day after school.

Amy and I were perfectly fine with the Paulie to Paul rebranding campaign, although Amy thought it was one more sign that Paulie—*Paul*—was growing up way too fast and would soon be out the door, off to college, into his own apartment, and only contacting us when he needed cash so he could take a year off to broaden his horizons backpacking across Europe with some girl named Natasha he met standing in line at Starbucks.

I said, "Babe, we have at least twelve more years with Paulie at home. He's not leaving for his freshman year in college just yet."

But maybe Amy was onto something. Twelve more years or not, the fact remained that in just one month Paul would be entering kindergarten—and that's where it all begins. Parental separation angst aside, Paul couldn't have been more excited about joining the ranks of all the "grown-up kids" he would see in the neighbor-

hood walking with their books as they made their way to school every morning.

His maturity star on the rise and playground influences notwithstanding, maybe Paul figured dropping the "ie" from his name would give him a bit of a credibility boost when he stepped into the classroom for the first time at St. Patrick's Episcopal Day School in early September. No matter what was going on inside that amazing six-year-old brain, Amy and I regularly thanked God for him, Daniel, and all the other blessings too numerous to mention in our lives. We had two healthy, growing boys who filled our lives with much joy; we couldn't have been any more grateful to God.

With Paul entering kindergarten for the first time in just a few weeks, our calendar was marked up with various dates and times related to his school schedule, as well as playdates and activities for Daniel. Most of the September days on the calendar had multiple events listed: first day of school, karate class, trampoline park, library visits, and on and on. But Thursday, September 19, had just one notation: CNMC, for Children's National Medical Center.

Just two weeks after his first day at school, Paul needed to take a field trip of sorts to Children's so he could undergo his third open-heart operation.

It was time for Dr. Richard Jonas to replace Paul's donated baby aorta, the homograph connector, with a newer, larger one that we hoped would carry him into his teenage years. During Paul's most recent angioplasty in December—*his seventh*—Dr. Slack confirmed what we already suspected: Paul and his current connector were both running out of steam.

Several times over the past six months, Paul had com-

plained of having chest pains and said he felt like he was running out of space around his heart. At various times throughout the spring and summer months, he also complained about having difficulty breathing, especially after running around with the other kids on the playground or at one sports activity or another. After he exerted himself, Paul's heart would sometimes be pounding in his chest like the pistons in a nitromethane-fueled dragster. These episodes were always frightening, not only for Paul but also for Amy, who increasingly found herself sitting off to the side with him as he clutched his chest and struggled to catch his breath.

Though not always rush-to-the-hospital emergencies, Paul's increasing complaints about how he was feeling were definitely evidence that the homograph he'd had in his chest for more than five years was losing its effectiveness and starting to fail because of all the stresses and strains created by Paul's growing body. And boy, was he growing! When Paul turned six years old in June, he weighed in at a hefty fifty-seven pounds and stood four feet two inches tall. Our pediatric cardiologist, Dr. Deneen Heath, was convinced Paul was going to wind up being at least six feet four or five and towering over Amy and me before we knew it. All great, but that rapid growth was really putting a strain on the connector in Paul's chest and just about everything else going on around his reconstructed heart.

As scary as some of those summer playground episodes were, Dr. Heath assured us Paul's heart would almost certainly not fail or go into any kind of cardiac arrest without us having major warning signs first. So even though he would often get winded or feel pressure in his chest, Dr. Heath told us Paul's body would self

regulate, and we shouldn't restrict him from running around or baby him in any way. Still, throughout the summer, Amy and I were very nervous and on high alert for the slightest sign Paul might be headed for trouble.

Once during the summer Amy took the boys to Trampoline Park, and after five minutes Paul's heart was ready to jump out of his chest, while younger Daniel could go for at least thirty minutes. Increasingly, Paul was getting tired more quickly than before, forcing him to take more breaks than the other kids he was playing with. Subsequently, the pace and duration of pretty much all of his physical activities had to be altered significantly throughout the spring and summer months.

I used to tell my friends across the country that D.C.'s heat in the dead of summer was akin to a St. Bernard dog constantly breathing down on you—wet, hot, and extremely sticky. With the city's legendary heat fast approaching came more concerns about how Paul would make out running around with his friends. Amy was extremely creative in the way she would adjust Paul's schedule without making too big a deal about it. Not wanting Paul to feel like he was missing out on anything or scare him in any way, Amy quietly changed his activities a little. Knowing Paul couldn't handle, say, an hour-long karate lesson, all his sessions became thirty minutes.

Throughout much of the summer Amy also became pretty much a helicopter mom, hovering around Paul and not letting him out of her sight for more than a few minutes at a time just in case there needed to be an unscheduled trip to Children's to have him checked out. Amy was as calm as any helicopter mom could be under the circumstances.

I, on the other hand, was a nervous wreck.

Sometimes calling Amy to check in during the day, what I heard on the other end of the line was, "Honey, don't worry, *but...*" Those words, of course, would always rocket my heart directly into my throat without passing go, and I would immediately start pacing around my office and yelling into the phone, "I am not worried. I am not worried!" Every time I received a call from Amy, before I picked up the phone I would imagine hearing, "We're at Children's. We need you here ASAP!" It was a nerve-racking time as we approached Paul's third open-heart operation.

Dr. Heath was incredibly helpful to us throughout this period. Paul's cardiologist pretty much from the beginning, Dr. Heath is truly an amazing woman. Not only smart as a whip about everything to do with pediatric cardiology, she could easily write a textbook on the topic of doctors and bedside manners. Dealing regularly with stressed-out parents worried sick about their children with heart disease, Dr. Heath always has a smile on her face and a tremendously calming effect even in the midst of some very scary moments.

We were very fortunate to have Dr. Heath as Paul's pediatric cardiologist for a lot of reasons. For one, she almost didn't make it into medicine at all.

Her father, a successful Wall Street real-estate type, wanted Deneen to do something entirely different, telling her, "Why don't you go into business and make something out of yourself?" Luckily for us, Deneen's first encounter with Economics 101 at Princeton University didn't turn out too well, so she circled back toward medicine. Seeing how caring she was with small children, Deneen's mother told her she should be a pe-

diatrician. Upon hearing that, once she was actually in medical school, Deneen, of course, tried everything she could *not* to be a pediatrician. She decided she wanted to be an orthopedic surgeon because that was what men did.

But as fate would have it, when Deneen did her required training in pediatrics, she absolutely fell in love with the children and had to admit her mom was right all along. After deciding to focus on children's health, Dr. Heath zeroed in on cardiology because she found the interactivity of the heart, lungs, and arteries— "plumbing and electricity," as she calls it—absolutely fascinating. Also, seeing all those stressed-out parents dealing with their children's heart issues, Dr. Heath liked the idea of being able to help families for months, sometimes years, holding parents' hands "through the entire journey," as she would often say. Having Dr. Heath by our side throughout our journey over the past six years had been a complete blessing that made our experience at Children's, if not pleasant, at least infused with a great measure of hope, optimism, and always with an ample supply of her contagious laughter.

One day early in the summer, after an episode during which his heart was racing and he was experiencing chest pains, Amy decided to talk to Paul about how we had a plan to get him all fixed up. She sweetly and softly spoke to him about how, after his upcoming surgery, he would be able to run faster, his heart wouldn't beat so fast, and he would be able to stay on that trampoline as long as he wanted. With his heart racing and still in a fair amount of discomfort, Paul looked at Amy and pointed both his thumbs high in the air while saying, "Two thumbs up. That would be great!"

Amy said it was a nice moment and reinforced her impression that as traumatic as these open-heart surgeries were, Paul understood the need for them and trusted everyone around him who was working hard to keep him healthy for the trampoline park, the playground, the soccer field, and all the other good things this life has to offer a six-year-old boy.

All through Paul's little-boy-growing-up years we knew this third open-heart surgery was on the horizon, but as the day got closer the stress monsters started paying their normal visits, only this time with much more intensity than five years ago. Amy was once again having a round of her really bad headaches, and when I was able to get any sleep at all, it was normally accompanied by very dark and recurring dreams about funerals and death.

Concerned about the dark thoughts and specifically the graphic nature of the funeral dream, I sought help from my local parish priest, Monsignor Peter Vaghi of the Little Flower Parish in Bethesda. Monsignor Vaghi, a former lawyer quite well known in legal and spiritual circles in D.C., was highly sensitive and very helpful to me throughout this time, praying with me and helping me work through the issue.

Another individual who helped me a lot during this time was a friend from Katy, Texas—Randy White. Not the Hall of Fame Dallas Cowboy tight end and linebacker of the same name, my Randy White happened to be a Southern Baptist preacher who always seemed to have the right words of encouragement and counsel when I needed them most. Often, Randy would send me e-mails with simple and meaningful prayers that helped me to stay focused and spiritually strong for everything we were facing with Paul.

With a Catholic monsignor in the heart of Washington and a Southern Baptist pastor in a small Texas town both regularly praying for me, not only did I feel fair and balanced in the spiritual resources department, I considered myself completely blessed that I had wonderful and caring people in my corner and watching my back during some very challenging days.

Even though Amy and I had been through this open-heart scenario twice before with Paul's earlier surgeries, I think the increased difficulty we were both having this time around had to do with the fact Paul was now able to talk to us about what was going on with him. Paul was older, and the way we talked to him about the operation had to make sense on his level. Unlike the previous surgeries when he was still a baby and not able to talk to us about what he was thinking or feeling, this time Paul had a lot on his heart and mind that he definitely wanted to express.

Amy and I therefore spent a fair amount of time talking to Paul about the surgery and doing our best to try to get him to buy into the idea that it was really a good thing and he shouldn't be too freaked out about any of it. Scared was fine, but not too scared. Sad, even worried, was okay, but not to the point of being depressed. To get him to a safe, calm place, Amy and I were constantly talking to Paul about all the great things he would be able to do after this surgery was behind him. We kept trying to paint a positive, uplifting picture for him. Not obsessively so, but whenever we could do so naturally—before bedtime, on a walk around the neighborhood, before school, or whenever it seemed like the right time to bring it up.

Apart from the way we were talking to Paul about the upcoming operation, unlike the previous surgeries when he was a baby, six-year-old Paul now had serious thoughts and feelings he could communicate to us. And it seemed like every day presented us with a new round of difficult questions about his heart and specifically what would be happening to him during surgery. One day early in the summer I woke up to, "Daddy, could I die from my surgery?"

Like anyone in that situation, I was completely thrown. I didn't want to be an elusive politician trying to squirm out of answering a difficult question, but I found myself stalling for time till I could come up with the right words. Eventually I said, "Buddy, we all could die anytime. But I am convinced you are going to have a long, healthy life. And in just a few weeks you are going to be running faster and jumping higher than you ever have before. New superpowers are coming to your heart," I said. Paul looked at me and smiled.

"Cool, Daddy!"—with two thumbs up again.

Even with all the tough questions from Paul, it wasn't as though the entire experience was totally new for him. After all, every morning when he woke up he could see the huge scars from two previous surgeries that ran directly down the middle of his chest, daily reminders that he was a little different from the other kids he played with. Amy and I both worried about those scars. What did he think about them, really? Kids being kids, what kind of grief would they cause him through the years? To Amy and me, those scars were beautiful because they represented life and the fact that Paul's heart had been fixed. But to a six-year-old mind—we just weren't sure what he thought about all that.

Trying to minimize the spells of darkness from descending and to keep everything as upbeat as possible, just a few weeks before the surgery Amy and I decided to take the boys to Florida for a family vacation. Both sets of grandparents have homes in Naples, so it would give the boys an opportunity to spend time with them while we tried our best to sit in the sun, romp in the waves, and think about anything other than intensive care units for a few days. One day while we were out by the pool we saw an older man sitting in a nearby hot tub with a big scar on his chest. He clearly had had heart surgery, and Amy said to me, "I wonder if I should bring Paul over to talk to him?"

"Yes! Good idea," I said.

So Amy got Paul and they walked over and introduced themselves to the man with the scar. I also went over to talk to the man who, coincidentally, was from Amy's hometown of Chicago and also a Fox News watcher.

Amy told the man we wanted to introduce ourselves to him because our son had had two open-heart surgeries, seven angioplasties, and was getting ready to have his third open-heart operation in just a few weeks.

"We saw your scar and thought Paul would think that was really cool," Amy said.

Getting a good look at the man in the hot tub, Paul said, "Wow! How did you get your scar?"

"Well, I have had two open-heart surgeries, too!" the man replied.

"Really?" Paul said. "Do you have more coming?"

"I hope I am done," the man said.

"Well, I have one coming up," Paul informed him matter-of-factly.

"I bet you are going to be A-OK. You are going to be just fine," the man told Paul.

Paul said, "Yeah, I think so, too."

Then, transforming himself into the grand inquisitor, Paul started asking the man specific questions about his scar, exactly how he got it, and how his heart felt after his operations.

The man said, "I still have a pacemaker in there."

"What's a pacemaker?" Paul asked.

The man in the hot tub tried his best to explain to a six-year-old exactly what a pacemaker did. After he was done with his explanation, Paul asked him, "So you have wires in your body?"

"Yeah. I have wires and a little machine in there in case my heart doesn't work the right way," he replied.

"Wow! You are a robot," Paul excitedly shouted.

After a little more discussion about the similarities in their chest scars, the man told Paul, "Your scar looks great!"

"Your scar looks great, too!" Paul replied.

Then Amy added: "Chicks dig scars."

I don't think the "chicks dig scars" comment had much of an effect on six-year-old Paul one way or the other, but his new scar-bearing friend seemed to enjoy it very much.

Although it was a fairly tense time for the family, Amy and I tried our best to keep things light as we got closer to September 19. The original date for the surgery was the 18th, but we were informed that citizen Dr. Richard Jonas had received a court notice saying he needed to report for jury duty that day. I had no idea what we would do if Dr. Jonas got selected for a trial, but as I was already so up to my eyeballs worrying about things I had little or

no control over, I decided there was no more room on my worry list for even one more item. In fact, looking on the bright side, we realized the nineteenth happened to be Paul Hills's birthday. We decided to take the date change as a good sign and move on.

Whether the surgery was on the eighteenth or the nineteenth, Amy and I weren't particularly thrilled that Paul would need to be pulled out of school for a couple of weeks after having just gotten there and met all his classmates for the first time. But with flu season approaching, the doctors wanted to perform the operation sooner rather than later. Fighting off germs and infection is critical when dealing with open-heart patients. And for children and adults, picking up a bacterial infection can be fatal to those undergoing highly invasive surgeries. It was a balancing act, because if we waited till the spring, there was a possibility the homograph might not last, not to mention the fact that Paul would continue having chest pains and breathing issues throughout the fall and winter months.

Even though Amy and I were complete basket cases and constantly second-guessing all the decisions we made about the timing of the surgery, Paul seemed to be pretty much taking everything in stride. Knowing he was having difficulty keeping up with the other kids, one day out of the blue Paul told me he was looking forward to being able to go to sleep then wake up and have his heart all fixed.

Another day he told me another reason he wanted his operation was because he would receive a lot of attention from people, get several gifts, then when he got home from the hospital he would be able to run faster, go swimming, and be able to jump on the trampoline

as long as Daniel. His chest might hurt a little bit, he said, but that was okay with him if it meant he would get better.

Wow! Where did this kid come from—*really*?

No doubt about it. Paul Francis Baier, aka Paulie, had definitely earned the right to have his "ie" retired and hoisted up into the rafters at the top of any arena in America during his induction ceremony into the Little Boy Hall of Fame.

It was a tough couple of weeks in Washington. Everyone was on edge for one reason or another.

The House of Representatives was working on a short-term spending plan to keep the government from running out of money. But the bill had a controversial provision in it that would defund President Obama's signature health care plan, also known as Obamacare. So from one end of Pennsylvania Avenue to the other, the town was completely tied up in knots. It really seemed as if both sides were ready to take this gigantic game of fiscal chicken all the way to the brink this time and let the government shut down. The financial markets were nervous about the standoff, and there was renewed talk about America's tenuous credit rating and what would happen if the government closed for business and defaulted on its obligations.

Along with the political intrigue of the possible shutdown, Monday, September 16, brought horrific news to the entire D.C. area when a deranged shooter murdered twelve people in a senseless act of violence at Washington's Navy Yard. The images of grieving family

members trying to deal with their loss just broke your heart as you imagined what they must be going through as they tried to make sense of it all. There was, of course, no sense to be made of it. Being paid to report the news, my job is to get the facts out there and keep my personal emotions out of it, but sometimes, I have to admit, that is extremely difficult to do, especially if there are children involved.

Despite the sadness and craziness of the week, Amy and I did our best to maintain as much normalcy as we could as the hours clicked down to Paul's surgery. My usual postwork routine was to try to get home as soon as I could after *Special Report* each night so I could help get the boys to bed. Racing out of the studio after signing off the air each night, I could usually be home in time for toothbrushing, reading one book, bedtime prayers, and lying down with Paul as he fell asleep.

Just like I used to do with my Catholic high school uniform at the end of the school day back in the suburbs of Atlanta, each night when I got home I would typically race in the door, take off my suit jacket, rip off my tie, kick off my shoes, and race upstairs to be with the boys. Paul seemed to enjoy my postwork ritual as much as I did, and one night, after complaining that his feet were hurting, he spontaneously added a new component to the mix—rubbing his feet.

Now the end-of-the-day activities included some serious foot rubbing before Paul could get to sleep. While he talked nonstop about his day at school, I found that after just a few minutes of rubbing his feet, Paul would be out cold. It got to the point where as soon as I would walk in his room he would immediately ask, "Daddy, can you rub my feet tonight?"

I remember thinking this might have to do with all the therapuetic touching Amy did when Paul was in the hospital for his first operation; all the times she held him through the wires and the tubes—rubbing his hands and feet as she sat with him in the chair next to his medical bassinet. I thought, "Now it's my turn!"

Some nights when it was impossible to make it home before bedtime, Amy would tell Paul that she could perform the foot rubbing until Daddy got there. I got a big kick when Amy reported to me one night that Paul matter-of-factly informed her, "You can rub my feet, but Daddy's really the best at it."

Before the foot rubbing would begin, bedtime prayers would normally be said, with us remembering each member of our family, then all the other people Paul's six-year-old mind decided needed the Lord's help. We'd thank God for all the blessings he had given us, and then we would ask for a peaceful and restful night of sleep. Not wanting to focus too much on the upcoming surgery, I would try to steer the prayers in the direction of asking God to keep us all healthy. Before long, Paul could see through that and started adding, "And Lord, please help the doctors fix my heart so I can run faster and jump higher." Eyes closed in the darkness of Paul's bedroom, I would smile as I said, "Amen."

With Paul's surgery set for early Thursday morning, I debated whether to take off work Wednesday. After talking to Amy, we decided it would be better for me to work since Paul would be busy with presurgery appointments and friends stopping by throughout the afternoon to visit. I compromised and spent the morning and part of the early afternoon at Children's while Paul had his blood drawn and X-rays taken. On the night before the

surgery, my plan was to slip out of the bureau the second we were done with *Special Report*.

Late in the afternoon we learned the network had secured an exclusive interview with Syrian president Bashar al-Assad on the topic of chemical weapons and his country's ongoing civil war. That interview, fed in from Damascus very late in the day, quickly became the basis for an extended, two-hour edition of that evening's *Special Report*. Instead of being able to leave right at 7:00 p.m. as planned, I had to stay in the bureau well into the evening. So much for my plans to skip out early that night. The days leading up to Paul's third open-heart operation were extremely busy to say the least.

Paul was scheduled to go into Children's early Thursday morning, and given how social media communication had changed from the days of Paul's first open-heart surgery five years before, during the week I sent out several tweets about Paul's operation. Those short messages instantly generated hundreds of prayers and good wishes for our family, which was touching, inspiring, and completely humbling.

I still intended to send out a longer, old-fashioned e-mail to our family and friends so I could give all our prayer warriors more details about what was going on. But because I had been so backed up with the news of the week, it took me forever to get around to it. Eventually I wrote the e-mail as I sat in the hospital waiting room just as Paul's operation was beginning. After five years, I felt like one of the Blues Brothers trying to get the band back together for a big comeback concert just as the stage lights were coming up.

September 19, 2013, 12:07 PM, Thursday
Subject: It's been a while

Family and friends,
It's been a while since I have written one of these e-mails.
Some of you already know today is Paulie's third open-
heart surgery—his last was five and a half years ago. Since
that time, he's added a brother, Daniel, who is his best
buddy and playmate. And Paulie, who now tells all of his
friends he likes to be called Paul, has become a real char-
acter.

Last night we laughed hysterically as we had a dance party
in his bedroom before bedtime. But the real belly laugh-
ing happened when he blurted out, "Daddy, you have a big
booty!" He's right, of course, and he could have said what-
ever he wanted to as far as I was concerned. This morning
he gave his brother Daniel a kiss and a hug before leaving
for the hospital. Daniel, who is usually talkative, too, was a
little quiet and looked a little sad. At three, he knows what's
going on with his big brother.

On vacation in Florida a few weeks ago, Daniel took a plas-
tic stethoscope and gave Paul a pretend checkup. He said,
"Paulie, I know your heart is broken, but I will fix your heart
right here so you don't have to go to surgery, okay?" Daniel
proceeded to give Paul a thorough exam.

Just before I started writing this e-mail, the pager I'm wear-
ing beeped: "Surgical update: Paul was placed on bypass
at 10:31 a.m. He is doing fine." That means we are about
three hours away from seeing Paul in the Cardiac Intensive
Care Unit.

Dr. Richard Jonas, one of the best pediatric heart surgeons in the world, is replacing what's called a conduit, a donated aorta that connects his right ventricle with his pulmonary artery. Long story short, it doesn't grow with Paul and he is growing like a weed—100th percentile in height, 70th percentile in weight (the stats pediatricians use to compare kids to the average). So it's time to get a new one. It's the third family that has lost a loved one and donated the organs so Paul could live. Think about that for a minute.

Paul has been a real trouper this surgery. He's embraced it. We talked to his kindergarten class the other day about what this surgery is all about and how long Paul will be gone. We were really fortunate that his cardiologist, Dr. Deneen Heath, came in as well to explain things to the kids. By the end of our little talk, Paul was taking questions from his classmates.

Q: "Do you have to get shots?"

A: "Yes, and I cry a little, but not much."

Q: "Do you have to take medicine?"

A: "Yeah, and it's pretty yucky, but I take it."

Perhaps sensing the discussion about taking medicine might have been a bit of a downer for his five- to six-year-old audience, Paul decided to switch it up a little when he said to the class: "So, do you want to see my scar?" At which point, he lifted up his shirt and showed the entire class his scars from the first two surgeries.

Then he said, "Last question."

Paul was essentially running his own press conference! One little girl raised her hand. Paul called on her and she asked, "When can we eat the donuts that your mom brought in for us?"

That question was a big hit and pretty much ended the news conference.

The pager just beeped again: "Surgical Update. Paulie is still on bypass and doing fine. Please be around the waiting room in one hour for another update."

So far, so good.

This morning Paul was consumed with the movie he was watching on an iPad—the animated flick Hero. With headphones on, he was oblivious to a lot going on, which was good. The anesthesiologist gave him some medicine to drink (which Paul accurately described to his classmates as "pretty yucky").

Eventually, we coaxed him to drink it, in what I'm sure sounded to the other presurgical bays as a fraternity party where members are trying to get a pledge to drink a shot of something. But the promise of a new bike as a reward when he's all done with this probably doesn't pop up in too many fraternity parties.

The medicine eased him. Then I held Paul on my lap with my arms around him, and he sucked in the anesthesia. He slowly went to sleep. I laid him on the table, we gave him

a kiss, and then we walked out. Amy and I shared a few tears, took some deep breaths, and came here to the waiting room, waiting anxiously for the next beep or buzz for some update.

The last time I wrote an e-mail like this was for Paul's seventh angioplasty in December. During the overnight stay after that, I was sleeping on the couch next to Paul's bed. He woke up in the middle of the night, and out of the blue he asked me, "Daddy, why do I have to do all of these things? All of these heart things—and all of my friends in school don't have to do it?"

That question hung there in the air for a little while . . . and I scrambled to think.

I said, "Buddy, because God has a plan for you. You are going to do amazing things in your life. He's got big plans for you. But he wants to test you first to see if you're up for it. And you're passing the test. You're doing great!" He just looked at me and said, "Okay, Daddy. I love you" and then turned over and went back to bed.

I do a lot of ad-libbing on air, but that was one of my better efforts. Now, as we wait for the next beep, we know God DOES have a plan and we're trusting that Paul, the fighter, is fitting right into it.

Thank you all for your prayers and good thoughts.

Bret and Amy

Based on all the tweets and e-mails coming my way throughout Paul's surgery, the prayers and good thoughts from all over the country seemed to have the effect we'd hoped for. After several hours Paul emerged from his third open-heart surgery like a champ and was resting in his room in the Cardiac Intensive Care Unit. Once again Paul was receiving some pretty amazing care from the doctors and nurses looking after him in the CICU.

One of the things that has really helped us through our experiences at Children's over the past six years has been the fact that so many of the same doctors and nurses tending to Paul have been there the entire time. That kind of continuity of care is unique and has been a total blessing in our lives.

Dr. Richard Jonas has performed all of Paul's heart surgeries going back to July 2007. Dr. Michael Slack has done six of Paul's seven angioplasties. Dr. Gerard Martin, the cardiologist who first showed up at Sibley to check on Paul when he was one day old, was still the head of Children's cardiology department. Dr. Kurt Newman, who performed the surgery on Paul's stomach in the summer of 2007, was now CEO of the entire hospital and has been a tremendous help to Amy and me over the years. Dr. Deneen Heath has been Paulie's cardiologist from almost the beginning of our time at Children's. In fact, on that first day at Sibley when Dr. Martin diagnosed Paul, the first person he called at Children's to get ready for Paul's transfer was the cardiologist on call that day, Dr. Heath.

Those five, and any number of other doctors and nurses at Children's, have been with us the entire journey, all vital and essential parts of Team Baier. That we

know them personally and they are all plugged in to the intricacies and nuances of Paul's heart always gives us an extra level of comfort whenever we are at Children's.

Not only do they have institutional knowledge about Paul's case, they are, without a doubt, all tops in their field. They are also wonderful people to deal with and have sincere compassion, sensitivity, and affection for our son, which is icing on the cake.

By the time of Paul's third surgery, Amy and I had started helping Children's with a few charitable events now and then. The folks at Children's even asked me to MC the hospital's annual fund-raising gala a few times, which I was thrilled to do. Along with Amy's folks, the Baier-Hills family had also been privileged to assist Children's with a few financial gifts along the way. What other response could we possibly have to the people who gave us our son back and offered our entire family a new lease on life?

To show our appreciation for all they had done for us, we had no choice but to join Children's team and be available to them whenever, wherever, and however they needed us. They had been such a vital part of our family for the past six years, we were compelled to become part of the unofficial team at Children's for the rest of our lives—or at least until someone told us to go away. And not just part of that team; we were all in.

Fighting heart disease is much more like running a marathon than a sprint; it is almost as if we are all part of the same relay team making our way around the track, handing the baton off to the next runner as we make our way to the finish line, and combining our efforts to battle pediatric heart disease. Also part of that great team effort over the years have been all the great folks outside the hospital who have been with us every step of the way:

Dear family and friends,

Thank you for your prayers and good wishes. They worked—and then some!

The last e-mail I sent you was written from the surgery center waiting room as Paul was heading into his third open-heart surgery. Postsurgery, there were definitely some sleepless nights in the Cardiac Intensive Care Unit, with beeps from the monitors triggering more heavy medicine; more beeps and concern about his lungs and shallow breathing; more beeps and worries about his high blood pressure.

A parent can make himself/herself crazy looking at those monitors, worrying about what beep will be next. But we had a feeling from the start Paul was going to power through recovery. Every picture we took of him—even at the beginning when he was still filled with drugs—he managed a smile. Every one!

As the days ticked by, the smiles got bigger. When we were moved to the heart and kidney floor (out of intensive care), I pushed the couch next to his hospital bed to sleep close to him, rubbing his back as he fell asleep and then holding his hand that was still wrapped in tape with an IV coming out of it (negotiating wires and tubes at bedtime is a challenge).

I definitively knew Paul was back to himself when at 3:00 a.m. he turned to me and said, "Daddy, this hospital stuff is boring." At which point I said, "Yes, buddy, it is. Let's watch another Scooby Doo on my iPad." So at 3:10, he smiled and gave me a kiss as Freddie, Daphne, Velma, Shaggy, and Scooby headed out on their next adventure. We didn't make it to the demasking of Blackbeard's ghost before Paul was back asleep. Well before the ever-present "I would have gotten away with it too, if it wasn't for you meddling kids!" Paul was breathing deep, and all the vital signs on the monitor were looking A-OK.

Paul lit up the most when his friend Alice Caroline came by for a visit. He perked up and laughed out loud for the first time (a great sign because laughing triggers coughs, and in open-heart surgery recovery coughing is key for clearing out the lungs, even though it's really painful in his chest that was just cut open days earlier). While his voice was weak, he talked about Halloween costumes and parties to come, as though the surgery had never happened. All with bright smiles.

Before long, Paul was walking around the nurses' station with a mobile monitor saying hi to everyone who walked by, a mini ambassador who was determined to walk his way out of the hospital. (We had told him the more he walked without feeling bad, the faster he'd be able to head home).

The biggest challenge was getting him to take medicine. He was making amazing progress. His vital signs were improving every day, but he had one more thing to check off the list before we could go home... he had to show the nurses he could take Advil and Tylenol by mouth before he could leave.

Paul has always had a serious problem taking medicine. It's like his taste buds just recoil even before it gets to his mouth, and then his mind kicks into full reject mode.

I know there have been tough negotiations between the Palestinians and the Israelis, the Russians and the U.S., Donald Trump and whichever business he's buying, but Paul was giving them a run for their money.

At one point, I was standing next to the nurse saying, "Okay, we're going to count backwards from 10 and then you are going to chug this medicine. "Ten, nine, eight." And Paul yelled, "WAIT!!! WAIT!!! What about starting at one hundred?"

We went through every flavor produced before we came upon the chewable grape versions of both medicines—and with a lemonade or Gatorade chaser—he could take it and keep it down. Success!

As hard as it was to believe, just five days after his third open-heart surgery, Paul was discharged. We had something to do first, though.

Two days earlier, when Paul was still in intensive care, Dr. Jonas introduced Amy and me to another couple. Dr. Jonas said, "In all my years of doing this, your two children have some of the most complex hearts I've seen, and as unique and rare as they are, they're almost exactly the same." He told us the complexity was a 12 out of 10 for both.

This family's baby boy, who was now five months old, had had two other surgeries at another hospital and then, after not seeing an improvement in his health, these parents reached out to Dr. Jonas. The baby was heading to his third major surgery in his short five-month-old life, a life that had been spent almost exclusively in the hospital.

We shared our stories about how we managed things, about how amazing Dr. Jonas is, and about the things that helped us get through: prayers, keeping healthy, being there for each other, and visualization.

For Amy, it was imagining Paul running around on the beach and playing in the sand. For me, seeing him walking down the first fairway with me and starting a round of golf. The couple, teary, nodded at each other knowingly. We gave them a hug and said we'd check in soon.

Now, before we left the hospital, we decided to bring the little boy some gifts: Cookie Monster, Handy Manny, and Spider-Man balloons Paul had been given and a little teddy bear.

We walked to his room in CICU, with Paul leading the way. The boy had taken a turn and wasn't there. They were prepping him for surgery early. His father was there, shaken and sad. He was appreciative of the gifts and said he would make sure his son saw them when he got out of surgery and woke up.

We gave him a hug, knowing that they were starting the scary journey again, a journey this boy had been through two times before and a journey Paul was walking away from after just five days in the hospital.

Walking out of the room, all three of us holding hands, Paul said these words:

"That daddy looks really sad and scared for his boy. We should pray for that family. We should pray for that boy."

Amy and I looked at each other with a loving look, both saying at the same time to Paul, "We should, Paul, and we will, every night."

And we did. And we have—each bedtime.

At the end of that week, after being home, Paul went back into his class for a short time. He talked to his kindergarten classmates about his surgery, thanked the kids for their cards and presents, and essentially held another news conference, taking questions and again lifting up his shirt, this time to show them his NEW scar.

At my work, another special thing was happening. I take the Special Report staff to dinner every so often for Idea Dinners, to kick around ideas about how to improve the show in some way. They came up with Special Report Gives Back, an effort to raise money or give time as a show to the local community in some way for charity.

The last dinner in August, with Paul's surgery looming sometime in September, they decided to make raising money for Children's National their first Special Report Gives Back, which humbled me.

So with my staff running point, Amy and I committed to be a part of the Race for Every Child, the first annual 5K run/walk for Children's on the National Mall the first weekend in October.

We weren't sure if we would be able to attend the race. Frankly, we didn't know if Paul would be up for going downtown to watch other kids run or walk while he couldn't. Little did we know that because of Paul's amazing recovery he would want to and would be able to walk in the 5K.

So there we were, all donning our race T-shirts early on a Saturday morning... alongside an amazing turn out from Special Report and the Fox D.C. bureau. Our three-year-old, Daniel turned to Paul and said, "I'm running with Daddy, you walk with Mommy."

Not that we let the three-year-old decide, but he did. When Daniel said he'd "run with Daddy," it was in a stroller. So I ran with Daniel as he told me from his perch what songs to play on my iPhone, and Amy and Paul started walking next to one of Paul's school friends and his mom.

Daniel ran the last 20 yards with me as we crossed the finish line pushing the stroller, and we waited for Paul and Amy. Amy said that a few times Paul got tired and she put him on her back. But he quickly wanted back down to keep walking.

And after a while I could see them in the distance walking up to the finish line, Paul proudly strolling and holding Amy's hand. The woman on the microphone for

Children's National saw Paul approaching, and over the loudspeaker she said, "Here comes Paul Baier—just seventeen days ago he had his third open-heart surgery at Children's, and today he's crossing the finish line after walking 3.1 miles!"

A huge cheer erupted all over the square. Paul's smile broadened from ear to ear. Daniel screamed, "Yay, Paulie!" I was snapping pictures but I didn't know if they were coming out because tears were streaming down my face.

I looked at Amy and she was crying, too, as Paul stepped across the finish line. Three weeks and four days after I wrote the last e-mail in that surgery center waiting room our son was walking proudly across the finish line of a 5K raising money for the hospital and the doctors and nurses who have saved his life more than once.

It was powerful. We are blessed—truly blessed. The event raised 700 thousand dollars for the hospital.

As gratifying and glorious as that finish line was, unfortunately, it's not the end of our race.

Paul may have more angioplasties (or tune-ups as his doctors call them). He may have another surgery eight to ten years from now or, if we're lucky, technology may improve to a point that he might indeed have had his last open-heart surgery. Time will tell.

But we're not dwelling on all of that right now. We're doing our best to focus on living and celebrating every smile!

Thank you for your thoughts and prayers—they truly helped us through the toughest hours and the darkest days.

Our race continues...

EPILOGUE

Washington, D.C.—January 6, 2014—6:58 p.m.

"...As always, thank you for inviting us into your home tonight and for every night over the past five years. That's it for this Special Report, *fair, balanced, and still unafraid."*

After my sign-off, the red lights on the studio cameras click off, stage manager, Mary Pat Dennert shouts "Clear!" and my 1,306th *Special Report* is history.

As I fully expected, tonight's show was extremely lively and filled to the brim with a wide range of interesting stories: chief national correspondent Jim Angle on the confusion about the Obamacare enrollment numbers; senior foreign affairs correspondent Greg Palkot on the rise of al Qaeda insurgents in Iraq; chief intelligence correspondent Catherine Herridge on Senator Rand Paul's class action lawsuit against the National Security Agency (NSA); chief Washington correspondent James Rosen on the U.S. Supreme Court and Utah's ban on same-sex marriages; and with tonight's last ever Bowl Championship Series (BCS) football game being played (Florida State vs. Auburn)—William La Jeunesse filed a story for us about the dollars and cents of amateur competition in America.

As always, the *All Star Panel*—Steve Hayes of *The*

Weekly Standard, Mara Liasson of NPR, and syndicated columnist Charles Krauthammer really brought their "A" games. We were fortunate also to have an on-set commentary from senior political analyst Brit Hume on the political and practical fallout from the upcoming congressional fight over extending unemployment benefits.

We ended tonight's program with a special segment marking my fifth anniversary anchoring the show. It was a fun bit of tape the staff put together that brought back a lot of fond memories. It reminded me how often we have taken the show on the road over the past five years—especially during election season.

Highlights on the tape included some snippets from a March 2010 interview I did with President Obama right before the big health care vote in the House of Representatives, as well as some of my 2011 interview with then presidential contender Mitt Romney on the eve of the GOP primaries.

The tape reminded me once again that the *Special Report* team of correspondents, producers, videographers, and editors is a very special group of people. They never cease to amaze me with their creativity and problem-solving skills—sometimes just seconds before that red light comes on.

A bit of superstition perhaps, but thirty seconds before we go on the air every night, I always say, "*Good show everyone.*" If I happen to forget, Mary Pat will clear her throat as a signal to make sure I remember. Doug Rohrbeck, *Special Report* executive producer and the voice in my head for the past five years, speaks to me in my ear from the control room through what's called an *IFB*. Doug quickly follows my "*Good show...*" with

a "*Good show!*" of his own usually followed by some addendum to whatever the running joke of the day has been.

After being together for five years we are all pretty much convinced the show will crash, burn and become an unmitigated disaster if I forget to utter my innocuous "*Good show everyone.*" One time I did forget and halfway into the show I lost my voice mid-sentence and actually shed a tear trying not to cough. After the segment, my mom e-mailed me to ask, "Were you getting emotional on that story or were you having throat problems?"

As much as it possibly can be around a fully operational newsroom on a very busy day, my *Special Report* anniversary created a bit of a festive atmosphere around the bureau today. In fact, midday, Amy and the boys made a surprise visit to help me celebrate with my colleagues. Three-year-old Daniel was particularly interested in the anniversary cake that happened to have a giant picture of me on it. "That's Daddy on there!" he laughed. Daniel is a really happy kid—a bright ray of sunshine who absolutely adores his older brother, Paul. He laughs all the time and is a real character. Daniel also happens to have a bit of a sweet tooth and the "*Daddy Cake*" was his latest target. James Rosen, a great friend, amazing correspondent and writer, insisted he have "*my head on a platter*"—cutting his own slice with surgical precision to achieve his goal.

Mark Twain, perhaps apocryphally, is often quoted as saying, "the key to success is getting started." Properly attributed or not, by all accounts I was bitten by the media bug and got my start in journalism at a very early age. As a young boy I remember pressing my face up

to the television set as I watched the national political conventions and those network reporters wearing their space-age looking headsets as they tried to navigate around the balloons and confetti on the convention floor.

How cool would that be to wear those funky looking headsets and romp around the convention floor like you owned the place interviewing one interesting newsmaker after another. Little did I suspect at the time that one day I would actually be one of those floor reporters—funky headsets and all.

And now—all these years later—anchoring the flagship political news program for Fox News Channel. Other than marrying the woman of my dreams, pursuing journalism as a career has proven to be the best decision of my life.

Being able to write, cover great stories, travel, and interview a long list of newsmakers over the years has been exhilarating. Often, when I travel around the country, folks come up to me at airports or on the street and ask me questions like, "What's the most interesting story you've ever covered?"—or—"What's *so-and-so* really like in person?" That second question is almost always about my good friend and syndicated columnist Charles Krauthammer. The answer—Charles is brilliant, funny, and a very caring person. He has also been a great source of strength to me throughout all of Paul's hospitalizations.

I don't know how others who are on television feel about it, but whenever I travel around the country I absolutely love meeting folks who watch the show. It is a blessing and never a bother. I greatly respect the relationship with the viewers and understand that it's a

personal decision for them to choose whom to watch every night. Being able to meet many of these folks during my travels is always a big treat for me.

No matter how busy or exciting working in television news is—*and it is*—the most important part of my schedule starts about an hour after the red lights on the studio cameras fade to dark. Even though I get to mix it up with VIP newsmakers just about every day of the week, and I could literally spend hours discussing the important issues of the day with the likes of Brit Hume, Steve Hayes, Mara Liasson, Charles Krauthammer, George Will, Juan Williams, Kirsten Powers, Chuck Lane, and Nina Easton—my real *All Star Panel* starts the moment I get home and can spend time with Amy and the boys. If I'm lucky, I can get home in time to read Paul a story and put him to bed. Daniel is usually already conked out by the time I walk in the door.

Tonight, when I walk into the house I open the door and Paul runs up to me hollering "Daddy!" I have been a general assignment reporter, bureau chief, national security correspondent, White House correspondent, and now a network anchor. But, for me—*Daddy*—is the best title in the universe. An added bonus tonight when I get home—Daniel is also still awake. He, of course, followed right behind big brother Paul yelling "Daddy!" too—copying Paul's every move. I immediately thought back about that big piece of anniversary cake that must still be coursing through Daniel's three-year-old system. Big hugs and then a kiss from Amy who followed the boys to the front door.

"Congrats again, babe. That's a real milestone," Amy said—referring to the five years at *Special Report.*

All fame is fleeting I suppose, because immediately

following Amy's congratulations, Paul turned the conversation to a much more important milestone around the Baier house.

"Daddy?" Paul asked, "when do you think I will lose my other front tooth and how much do you think the tooth fairy will give me for that one?"

Just two days ago, Paul—with Amy's help—yanked out one of his two front teeth. He didn't even cry—just yanked the thing right out. Despite the blood and the pain, Paul was determined to get his tooth out so he could get his hands on some of that tooth fairy cash he has been hearing so much about.

After all Paul has been through in his short life, I think he must have thought this tooth-yanking business was kid stuff—and he was on the job.

Lately there has been an ongoing family debate about just how much a front tooth was going for these days. I remember fifty cents under my pillow when I was his age, but Paul's friends at school apparently have discovered some higher dollar tooth fairies, and they are definitely colluding on the numbers. So, after a recent meeting of the tooth fairy committee, it was decided that a front tooth under the pillow of a six-year-old would probably be rewarded with six one-dollar bills. Hearing that, Paul was highly motivated to yank out more teeth ASAP.

Before long, Daniel, who at three really is *the* sweetest kid on the planet, said, "Daddy, I'm tired. Can *you* put me to bed tonight?" Paul quickly chimed in, "No Daniel! He's putting *me* to bed tonight!"—Paul's toothless enunciation a little less precise than we are used to.

"Here's the deal," I said. "I'll put you *both* to bed. But, Daniel has to go now and Paul is next. Mommy can start

Paul by reading a book and then I will come in." With that bit of bedtime choreography worked out, Daniel smiled and said, "Okay Daddy." Paul grimaced a little, but finally relented, "Okay, but hurry, Daniel. You need to go right to sleep, okay?" Daniel took the order in stride, "Okay, Paul." To his credit, Daniel did as his older brother instructed. The cake must have worn off and in about two minutes Daniel was fast asleep and breathing deeply.

I tiptoed out of his room and across the hall to Paul's room where Amy was wrapping up the last paragraph of the latest adventures of *Captain Underpants*. Paul laughed heartily at every potty term in the book, and you can imagine how many there are in a book entitled, *Captain Underpants and the Preposterous Plight of the Purple Potty People*. Amy kissed Paul and said, "Good night, pumpkin." Paul kissed her back saying, "Good night, Mama—I love you." "Love you too!" Amy replied, as she closed the door.

I climbed into bed next to Paul and turned off the light. The blue glow of his night-light illuminated Paul's face and I could see he was lying on his pillow with a big smile on his face. "Why are you smiling?" I asked. Paul looked at me and said, "I don't know." He paused and then said, "I love you, Daddy."

I said, "I love you too." Then we did what we did every night at bedtime. We prayed together.

"In the name of the Father, the Son, and the Holy Spirit, Amen. Dear Lord . . ."—I started. Then, suddenly Paul took over. With his hands together and his eyes closed, Paul prayed, "Dear Lord, thank you for a wonderful day with Daddy's work party and thank you for Mama and Daddy and Daniel and me. Please keep us

all healthy and please help my other tooth to come out soon—because I want it to."

I smiled in the darkness and added, "And Lord, thank you for all you have given to us and for watching over our family. We are truly blessed. Please be with those who need you most." Then Paul remembered, "Oh, and Lord, please be with those kids in the hospital who have surgeries coming up and are really sick. Make them better and make their families happy." I finished up the prayer with "We ask this in Your Name" as we said together—"*Amen.*"

There were many times right after Paul's last surgery when just hearing him say these prayers would make me tear up. Tonight, the prayers bring a grateful smile to my face. "Good night, Daddy. I love you really a lot," Paul said. "I love you really a lot too, buddy," I said, as I rubbed Paul's back until he too was breathing deeply like his little brother.

After three open-heart surgeries, seven angioplasties and a stomach surgery—and with at least one or two more open-heart operations to come—Paul is truly an inspiration to me. Even though he's only six, he has taught me a lot. He's made me a better dad, a better husband, a better anchor; he's just made me better. I hope his story can inspire others and provide comfort to those who are going through tough times. There's a reason why Paul is still with us and I truly believe this book is a part of it. God has a plan for him and our family is going to soak in and celebrate every moment of it.

ACKNOWLEDGMENTS

Although it has been a few years since I played competitive team sports, I am very fortunate to say I am still part of two Hall-of-Fame teams.

The first—the team of men and women of Fox News and specifically those who help get *Special Report* on the air every night. I am humbled by their daily commitment to excellence as they toil to make the show the best it can be night after night. My name might be built into the opening title graphics, but these dedicated professionals make up the show's foundation and are responsible for the great success we have had over the years. More importantly—they have been a great source of strength and support to Amy and me throughout all of Paul's surgeries and hospitalizations.

I would especially like to thank Fox News president and CEO Roger Ailes who saw something in me many years ago and plucked me out of local TV to work for Fox News Channel. Roger has never missed an opportunity to help me succeed, and for that I am forever grateful. Roger has also been incredibly supportive of me and my family throughout all of Paul's health challenges. Above all else, Roger values family—something I have seen firsthand time and again. And I value his

friendship and the example he has been in my life over the years.

A special thank you also to former *Special Report* anchor—now senior political analyst—Brit Hume, for his unwavering support, both personally and professionally. Brit's shared insights and concern for me and my family has meant more than he will ever know.

Another great team I am privileged to be part of are the doctors, nurses, staff and technicians at Children's National Medical Center in Washington, D.C. Until Paul was admitted for his first surgery in June 2007, Amy and I had never even heard of Children's. Now, not a day goes by without us thinking about the people there, their professionalism and the many kindnesses extended to the Baier family over the past seven years.

Special Heart details my overflowing gratitude to Drs. Richard Jonas, Gerard Martin, Deneen Heath, Michael Slack, and Kurt Newman and their colleagues.

To the hundreds of other unnamed nurses, doctors, and staff at Children's who are working every day to keep Paul—and all the other boys and girls—healthy and happy, I offer a heartfelt "Thank you" for your service and dedication.

I would also like to thank Jim Mills, writer and collaborator on this project. Jim's ability to capture my voice as we bounced copy back and forth, refining every last word, has been invaluable. What started a year and a half ago as an informal conversation with a friend and former colleague about one day working on a project together became a *real* book because of some great teamwork. My manager, Larry Kramer, and book agent, Claudia Cross, greatly helped to keep this project on track and get it across the finish line.

Lastly, and most importantly, Amy and I would like to thank those unknown parents, who, in their deepest moments of grief and despair, somehow found the grace to allow their child's organs to be donated so that others might live. On behalf of our son Paul—and all the other children who live and breathe because of your courage—our prayer is that the peace of God "which passes all understanding" will truly be yours forever. Thank you.

AN INTERVIEW WITH PAUL'S HEART SURGEON—DR. RICHARD JONAS

Bret: Dr. Jonas, this, of course, is not the first time I've said this to you. But, for the record: on behalf of the entire Baier-Hills family—I want to say a heartfelt *Thank You*. Your diligence and ongoing efforts to give Paul a second chance at life have been absolutely amazing. Just the other day Paul had basketball practice and while he was running up the court he turned to me and said, "Daddy, I can run faster now!" I said, "You sure can, buddy!" So, for that moment—and a thousand more just like it—a sincere *Thank You*.

Dr. Jonas: It's been my pleasure. I think I warned you right after the last operation—when we replaced that obstructed tube that was in there—Paul actually might have more energy than you really wanted. You may want to turn it down a bit. [laughter]

Bret: No. He's doing fantastic and we can't thank you enough! You've operated on Paul's heart three times now. Going back to that first operation in July 2007, I wonder if you can remember what you thought when you learned of his case—when you saw his chart for the first time?

Dr. Jonas: Well, Paul had a very complicated combination of problems. He really had four or five major problems with his heart. A lot of the operations that we do are modular—essentially one module on top of another on top of another. Paul was going to require a very complex operation because his problems sort of worked one against the other. That meant

that the design and the construction of his new heart was going to be pretty challenging. He also was just a newborn so we were dealing with fragile tissue. Even the tiny needles that we use for stitching blood vessels together make a big enough hole and newborn blood doesn't clot very well. So, with hundreds and hundreds of needle holes, you're looking at a risk of significant bleeding for a big, reconstructive operation like Paul needed. *Trepidation* would probably be the best term to describe how I felt as I looked at the challenging combination of problems that Paul had.

Bret: It was so complex. His heart was about the size of a walnut and you're reconstructing the entire thing.

Dr. Jonas: Well, we use a lot of magnification. It doesn't look like a walnut with a lot of magnification. So—you sort of step into a different world, and things don't seem as small once you're in there.

Bret: One of the reasons I wanted to talk to you today was so folks might get an idea about some of the advances in pediatric heart disease—pediatric heart surgery—over the years. Jumping right in: what has changed, even since Paul's first surgery to now?

Dr. Jonas: Well—really the biggest changes occurred in the late 1970s as I was just starting out in this field. Prior to that, operating on newborns with Paul's level of complexity would be quite impossible. He would not have survived.

Bret: No chance?

Dr. Jonas: He probably wouldn't even have been diagnosed as to what his real problem was before he would have passed away. In the late 1970s—a new medication came along—*Prostaglandin*. And that meant you could keep a child alive for at least a week or two—long enough to diagnose their problem. At that point we also didn't have diagnostic methods like *echocardiography*. It was in the late 1970s that

ultrasound techniques were developed so you could diagnose a problem with minimal invasion. You could just put a probe on the chest and begin to understand how complex the problem was. Those were huge developments when they came along in the late 1970s. That really opened the whole field of neonatal, newborn heart surgery, which was what Paul was able to benefit from.

There have also been other advances in the heart surgery field in the last ten to fifteen years. Unfortunately, they're in areas that don't really directly benefit Paul. The most important area has been in ventricular assist devices like Vice President Cheney had implanted in his chest. These new miniaturized electric pumps really revolutionized the care for someone who's got muscle failure—if the heart muscle is burned out because of repeated heart attacks. Occasionally you see that in a very young child who's developed a viral infection and the heart muscle just suddenly stops, or at least weakens so rapidly that they need support with a mechanical device. So ventricular assist devices have really advanced tremendously in the past ten to fifteen years.

Bret: What about developments in the whole area of understanding what actually causes congenital heart defects? Genetic or environmental factors?

Dr. Jonas: There's a lot of work going on in that exact area and we're going to know a lot more in probably another ten years or so. The human genome was only first fully analyzed about 2001 and it costs billions of dollars. Now you can do a whole human genome analysis for $1,000 or maybe a couple thousand dollars. There's just been an explosion of data over the past several years. Suddenly, we've got genetic information from lots and lots of people with heart problems. Trying to decode all of that data and figure out what change in that person's genome is responsible for a

particular heart problem (is extremely difficult). So, there's a massive amount of decoding going on right now. It's actually pretty confusing. I think we're in the stage of just having too much information and really not knowing how to interpret it. But it will (eventually) lead to a really good understanding of what causes congenital heart problems. Hopefully in the future this will lead to actually being able to eliminate congenital heart problems altogether.

Bret: We talked a lot about this in the book. But, Amy and I were completely blindsided by all this. That first day we were told Paul was perfect. Then just one day after he was born, Dr. Gerard Martin made the diagnosis of Paul's heart defects at Sibley Hospital...

Dr. Jonas: ...Though in some ways that (not knowing) can be a blessing in disguise.

Bret: True. Amy and I have talked a lot about that.

Dr. Jonas: It's stressful for families to know three or four months before their baby's born that they're going to be dealing with a heart problem. I mean, if they're very careful planners they can look beyond the stress and use the information to plan how they are going to deal with it—where they're going to go to have the surgery, who their surgeon's going to be, that sort of thing. But...

Bret: You know us too well...

Dr. Jonas: You and Amy were just remarkable. We have a lot of families who are hit with all that scary information at one time. They've been through the stress of pregnancy, the exhaustion of a delivery and then they are shocked to find out their child has a heart problem. But, I have to say—there has never been a couple like you and Amy. You guys were just so remarkable the way you took the information in, processed it, and were calm and considerate of the other families who were there, of the staff and really just loving and

comforting Paul in every way. It was truly—and this is a completely unpaid solicitation—I mean, that's truly from the heart. It was quite remarkable how composed and how well you dealt with what was a very stressful situation.

Bret: Thank you. I mean, it was a family there at Children's. It really was. We felt that way the entire time we were there. On another topic: have things changed since then in this whole area of early warning signs or diagnosis?

Dr. Jonas: Fetal echocardiography is really progressing. I mean it was only in the late seventies that echo machines were developed where you could put a probe on a baby's chest and you could see anything at all in terms of figuring out the heart problem. Getting good images when the ultrasound has to pass through the mom's abdominal wall through the uterus through the fluid. You have the baby moving around inside the amniotic fluid. It's really amazing that those ultrasound machines can give you good images now. That's where there has been a lot of advance in the last ten to fifteen years. We can even get fetal MRI scans that give you even more information than the echo and look at the baby's brain as well as the heart. So, advances in fetal echocardiography are still moving along.

Bret: Isn't there now an inexpensive simple oxygen test that can be done? A simple finger test of some sort?

Dr. Jonas: Yes. It's called a *Pulse Oximeter*. Fetal problems are missed if a baby is born like Paul was. It's even possible for a baby to go home from the hospital undiagnosed. Because while the baby still has the fetal circulation, it can take a few days before you get the transition to what we call a mature circulation.

Bret: So, in a sense, even though the heart is operating the wrong way—it's still pumping.

Dr. Jonas: Yes. And it's allowing a baby to stay alive. In

some circumstances, the only change is a very slight change in the oxygen level. A baby doesn't become really blue. Some babies will be really blue and get really sick. But others will stay relatively well and unless somebody is extremely well trained, has a really good eye for color change, they could miss the fact that there is a slight blueness. The child will leave the hospital and get really, really sick at home when they do have an abrupt change from the fetal circulation to the post-natal circulation. So, the *Pulse Oximeter* is a little machine that you put on a fingertip and can detect very fine changes in oxygen level. That's been a big advance in screening and helps to pick up kids who would otherwise be missed.

Bret: But, they're not yet mandated for hospitals to use right?

Dr. Jonas: Well, Dr. Gerard Martin's been very heavily involved with this together with the American College of Cardiology and other cardiology groups. It is something that's beginning to become the standard of care on a state-by-state, hospital-by-hospital level.

Bret: Along with being a surgeon and performing hundreds of complicated surgeries like Paul's and others every year, you're actively involved in various research projects at Children's. I'm wondering if you could give folks a sense of what you're up to?

Dr. Jonas: Well, the main focus of my research has been to try and optimize the development of the brain in kids who also have heart problems. In the early years of heart surgery, there were a lot of specific problems related to the heart and lung machine. A lot of pediatric devices we used on children in the early days were actually developed for adults. So, we would take a machine designed to support a 200-pound adult and connect it to a four or five pound baby. Needless to say, under those circumstances, the machines didn't work as well

as we would like. That's really the way things worked in the '50s, '60s. It wasn't until the 1970s that there were some early machines designed for bigger kids. It wasn't really until the 1990s, early 2000s that we started to get the equipment we needed for newborn heart surgery.

The organ that's most sensitive to the harmful effects of using a very big machine on a baby is the brain. You get tiny particles that can travel to the brain and block off blood vessels. This can cause strokes inside the baby's brain. In the early years of heart surgery this was a very big problem. Now there are very good filters and surfaces designed to avoid platelets and white blood cells clumping together and blocking off blood vessels and allowing us to minimize the inflammatory response to the heart and lung machine. The heart and lung machine is perceived by the baby's body as being a huge invader. So, when you send a baby's blood through plastic tubes the baby's body assumes this is a massive infection and you get a whole body inflammatory response.

The brain is developing very, very rapidly in the newborn and that inflammatory response affects particular cells within the brain. So, our particular focus in research right now is trying to figure out which cells are most sensitive to inflammatory effects and how can we potentially reduce those effects and even replace those cells that died because of the impact of the heart and lung machine.

Stem cell implants into the developing brain is also an area that we're just beginning to explore.

Bret: So, paint a picture, five, ten, twenty years down the road if you would. Look into your crystal ball and tell us what your field will look like.

Dr. Jonas: Well, I think in the very long term. I really don't know if we're talking twenty years or fifty years or 100 years. The whole genetic area is going to have the biggest impact.

There's no question that genetic factors have a lot to do with the development of heart problems. It's not hereditary. It's not as though you have heart conditions that are passed from one generation to the next. Usually, it's random. Congenital heart defects just suddenly pop up in families with no history of heart problems. We need to understand what it is about that genetic code that causes that to happen and what we can do to neutralize that change so it doesn't result in heart development problems. So, I think that's going to be the biggest area where we are going to see the greatest impact.

Ventricle assistic devices for kids are also going to be important. Right now there are no implantable assist devices for kids even though there are several for adults. Those will probably benefit mainly kids who are born with a single pumping chamber. Most people have two pumping chambers, one for the lungs and one for the body.

A lot of our most complex kids have only a single pumping chamber and they end up with an operation called the *Fontan Operation,* which doesn't give them a pump for the lungs. Blood gets through the lungs, but at higher pressure than it should. It backs up into the body a little bit in some kids and that can have bad affects on the liver, kidneys, intestines, and so on.

If you could implant a little tiny pump—just a little booster—then that would give all of those kids a much better quality of life. And there are already implantable battery systems, so you can charge the battery of an implantable pump-up just by laying a charger over it. You don't actually have to have wires coming out through the wall of the abdomen or the chest anymore.

Bret: Circling back to Paul's case. He's had three surgeries now. And it looks like he's going to have a fourth sometime in his teens.

Dr. Jonas: Yep.

Bret: We obviously try to pin you down all the time about exactly when you think that fourth operation might be needed. But, beyond that—is there anything on the horizon that could negate the need for that surgery or might change Paul's scenario going forward.

Dr. Jonas: Well, the entire area of growing replacement parts.

Bret: Stem cells?

Dr. Jonas: Right. That would definitely benefit kids like Paul because he had a coronary artery running right across the front of his heart in an unusual location. That was one of Paul's big challenges. We had to bridge over that coronary artery with a non-growing tube and we used a human artery with a valve in it from a child organ donor. Paul's outgrown them, of course. He's a lot bigger now than he was then. He was a newborn when he had his first operation. So, if we could use tissue engineering and stem cells to develop a growing tube so a newborn baby would take some of his own cells or maybe even stem cells from a family member.

Bret: Like cord blood cells?

Dr. Jonas: Yes, like stored cord blood that would potentially give you stem cells that could grow in a tube that his body wouldn't reject and would be able to grow with him. That would be another very big advance.

Bret: Couple more things. I know some folks would be interested in how you get ready for surgery. How you map it out. As you described to me before, you plan it out the night before. You see it. Describe that. And then you kind of sleep on it?

Dr. Jonas: I do. I really think that it's important the night before complex operations to allow your brain to think about it all through the night. It's actually quite helpful because the

sequence of these operations is really important. The exact order. I mean it's a little like potentially painting yourself into the corner of a room. If you don't do things in exactly the right sequence—A: it takes a lot longer and—B: you might actually have to take part of the operation down and get back to an area that requires additional suturing or additional implantation of a patch. So, we do have to think about time. There's a limited amount of time. We're stopping the heart. We're starving it of blood during the time we're operating inside of it.

Bret: It actually stops. You're stopping the heart. Putting the body on this machine. It's actually coming to a full stop?

Dr. Jonas: Right. The body is being supported with the heart and lung machine. So, the blood is pumping to the brain and to the kidneys but the heart itself has to stop because you're working inside it. So, the way we do that is to put a clamp across the main artery to the coronary arteries and the heart is now effectively having a massive heart attack, except we've cooled it down to a very low temperature and we've injected a chemical solution that paralyzes that muscle. Stops it consuming energy. And that gives you around about two to three hours when you can work safely inside the heart. So, you've got the stopwatch ticking. That's where you really have to plan it out. I've watched plastic surgeons—terrific plastic surgeons—re-do a flap, something complex, four or five times until they're completely happy with it. We don't have that luxury. We have to get it right the first time.

Bret: And then there's a point when you're undoing that clamp and you're ready to take him off the machine and that heart needs to start again.

Dr. Jonas: Parents often express to me that they're worried the heart won't start at all but it will always develop some activity. The question is that we want to see that it's going to

take the load—whether or not it's strong enough to take over from the heart and lung machine. So, the real critical time is when we transition from the heart and lung machine to the heart itself. How well will it take that load? That's really the key time. That's when we will hold our breath.

Bret: You have an amazing ability to explain things and be calm about it. You have an amazing bedside manner. These are kids that you've opened up. You deal with the kids and with the parents in the waiting room. How do you process all that? I mean, it's not the carburetor of a '57 Chevy that you're working on. You have to detach a little bit right?

Dr. Jonas: Yep. It's the paradox of surgery. You do have to be caring and empathetic but you also have to be able to switch off and detach and become a bit of a robot in a sense. I've been called "Iceman." I'm not sure how kindly that's been said by some people but it takes a certain personality type. We have many people interested in the field of pediatric heart surgery, but it does require a certain personality type to be able to master that detachment. Many, many very outstanding adult heart surgeons say to me that they would never try to do what we do. They just feel it's not in their make-up to do it. So, even within the field of heart surgery, pediatric heart surgeons are considered a little bit different.

Bret: But later when you see a kid who's been on that operating table graduate from college and write you a letter, or writes his college entrance essay on his or her experience or write you a thank-you note—or—you hear about a little boy running faster on the basketball court—that's gotta be pretty special.

Dr. Jonas: It really is. It's truly been remarkable that my career started almost the day that this field started because I started out just as *Prostaglandin* was being released and that

really allowed me to be part of the neonatal revolution. That totally changed pediatric heart surgery. So, (those kids) feel like my own kids really. They're graduating from college and getting married and writing letters to me and it's really an incredibly warm and rich experience to be able to feel like I've got this whole family out there—just like my own kids. You know, you go through the ups and downs and all the challenges. You remember some of those difficult times when you faced very serious challenges with the kids themselves and with their parents. To finally get them to that college graduation or their wedding day is really terrific.

Bret: Dr. Richard Jonas—Thank You.

SPECIAL HEART